Complications of Cataract Surgery:

A Manual

To Sarah and Mandy

Complications of Cataract Surgery:
A Manual

Bruce A. Noble BSc, FRCS, FRCOphth
Consultant Ophthalmologist and
Director of Anterior Segment Service,
United Leeds Teaching Hospitals
Senior Clinical Lecturer in Ophthalmology,
Leeds University Department of Surgery

and

Ian G. Simmons BVSc, MB, ChB, FRCS, FRCOphth
Consultant Ophthalmologist,
United Leeds Teaching Hospitals
Senior Clinical Lecturer in Ophthalmology,
Leeds University Department of Surgery

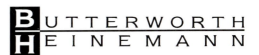

OXFORD AUCKLAND BOSTON JOHANNESBURG MELBOURNE NEW DELHI

Butterworth-Heinemann
Linacre House, Jordan Hill, Oxford OX2 8DP
225 Wildwood Avenue, Woburn, MA 01801-2041
A division of Reed Educational and Professional Publishing Ltd

ℛ A member of the Reed Elsevier plc group

First published 2001

© Reed Educational and Professional Publishing Ltd 2001

British Library Cataloguing in Publication Data
Noble, Bruce
   Complications of cataract surgery: a manual
   1.   Cataract – Surgery – Complications
   I.   Title   II.   Simmons, Ian
   617.7'42'059

Library of Congress Cataloguing in Publication Data

A catalogue record for this book is available from the Library of Congress

ISBN 0 7506 4799 X

Designed and typeset by Keyword Typesetting Services Ltd, Wallington, Surrey
Printed and bound in Italy

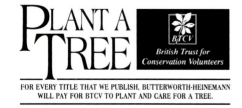

Contents

Preface

This book sets out to discuss and demonstrate a practical approach to the complications of cataract surgery and to weave into this ideas and ways of thinking to enable you to identify and handle these confidently. Complications can occur at any stage of the operation, but if recognized early can be handled and the surgery safely completed. We hope this straightforward book will give you the didactic advice and alternative techniques to help when you feel lost with a problem during or after an operation.

Every complication should be regarded as an opportunity to learn something new. The guidelines we suggest are simple and are entirely based on our lengthy experience as practising surgeons and surgical tutors. Having personally experienced every complication ourselves, and managed many more coming later for revision, we feel able to offer these solutions, some of which are novel while others are derived from the suggestions of greater surgical masters. They are mixed and melded together and presented in the hope that they will help you in specific situations or generally when thinking about your approach to cataract surgery.

Although we have written with aspiring surgical trainees in mind, we hope the book will also be of use to surgical probationers of every age. We stress the importance of the diligent application to seeing, learning and applying as wide a range of surgical techniques as possible. As the surgical repertoire becomes narrower, take the trouble to also learn the 'old ways' of operating too, even if these are in the wet-lab and on cadaver eyes. These efforts will be repaid handsomely during a long career in ophthalmic microsurgery. Surgical mastery is not readily attained, but being able to understand and cope with complications is a necessary step on the way.

There are many people to whom we owe a debt of gratitude as we submit this book for a wider readership. First, we are grateful to our teachers for giving us room to make mistakes and to mend them. Without support like theirs any surgical probationer would have given up long ago. The traditions of nurturing surgical ambitions require the ability to share enthusiasms and not to scorn when things go wrong.

Dr John Gibson, Consultant Anaesthetist at the General Infirmary at Leeds, gave freely of his time and experience as he wrote and argued his way through the chapter on anaesthesia. His interest in ophthalmic anaesthesia was aroused by the lectures and publications by Drs R.F. Hustead and R.C. Hamilton of the Gimbel Eye Centre and the University of Calgary. Their teaching has in part formed the basis of his text. He acknowledges his debt to these and many other published authors. His support during many long operating lists over the past 20 years has supported the surgery and training of many young ophthalmologists; we are grateful to him for his significant contribution.

We are grateful to our colleagues in the eye departments at Leeds General Infirmary and in Yorkshire for their helpful criticisms on this book during its gestation, and for reading the text to see whether we were drifting away from its purpose. Caroline Makepeace at Butterworth-Heinemann gave excellent support as we started out on this book and it is largely due to her enthusiasm that we continued until it was finished. Jack Kanski, FRCS, FRCOphth, that doyen of ophthalmic writers, gave us early and telling criticism that sharpened our minds to the new discipline of writing as opposed to operating. Michael Geale, our Ophthalmic Diagnostic Imaging Specialist (as medical photographers are now known) has taken all the photographs included in the text, and his understanding of what each photograph should show makes these pictures so special and useful. We are indebted to him and his skills.

Finally, we must thank our wives and families for their consistent support during the extended writing of this book. Their tolerance of the many nights and weekends spent away from them, talking, writing and reading, are added to the years of support given to us as we pursued our surgical careers. This book is dedicated to them.

Bruce Noble and Ian Simmons
Leeds

Introduction

The surgical removal of a cataract and its replacement with a synthetic implant (IOL) is the 'bread and butter' operation for the majority of ophthalmologists. It has a staggeringly high success rate and it is easy to forget just how much skill and training is required to achieve these outcomes.

In the developed world, the surgical removal of the crystalline lens is predominantly by phacoemulsification. The surgery is repetitive, and because of the high levels of success, low complication rates and ambulatory surgery, there is a real risk of the operation being perceived as trivial. Yet to produce such success rates, a constant need to operate to the highest standards is demanded. In spite of the apparently facile surgery (too many successes?) there remain many potential steps in the process where things can go wrong.

When something goes wrong, recognition of the fact is a primary requirement and opens the door for the appropriate management to start. The outcome of any complication will depend on what happened, how quickly the problem was recognized and the skill with which it was managed. This requires the thoughtful application of alternative surgical and medical treatments, which will contain the complication and allow the surgeon to finish the operation safely. If that operation is for the removal of cataract, the delicate tissues of the eye require the surgeon to have a clarity of approach and sureness of touch to limit damage and achieve restoration of sight.

Both phacoemulsification and extracapsular extraction of the lens (ECCE) involve completing a sequence of steps that follow in a logical order. The successful execution of each is the key to starting and completing the next. This is particularly true in phacoemulsification, where, if something goes wrong at an earlier stage, even something quite small such as a nick in the capsulorrhexis, difficulties at later stages are to be expected. The cascade of consequences can be serious.

A skilled and experienced surgeon will be able to perform each of these steps in a practised, almost automatic way. The need for such unconscious skills becomes crucial in more challenging cases and particularly when complications arise. Here the surgeon's concentration must be directed at the problem to hand and not distracted by anxieties such as how to use a particular piece of equipment or do a particular manoeuvre, e.g. 'How do I use a vitrector?' or 'How do I put in a stitch?'. However, the nature and

length of modern surgical training means that the knowledge of how to handle a complication may be only theoretical.

The difference between a good surgeon and an excellent one is practice. It has been said the difference between a professional musician and an amateur one is that whilst an amateur will practise until they get a piece of music *right*, the professional will practise until they *never get it wrong;* as professionals, we should aspire to the latter idiom. Each of the steps of cataract surgery justifies concentrated effort and rehearsal. When starting to operate, new surgical trainees should master the individual steps of the operation such as lens insertion or capsulorrhexis. Similarly, a more experienced surgeon should be able to use the equipment and handle the added challenge if a complication occurs.

The elegant handling of a complication will depend on containing the problem and carrying out the logical and timely manoeuvres. Having spotted the problem at an early stage, the surgeon must regain control and poise, and not go blundering on. Take time to quietly observe and plan a response. Then having planned what needs to be done, the surgical response can start. The surgical steps needed to repair the situation will depend on the complication. Again the limited surgical apprenticeship of modern training means that some of the manoeuvres may never have been either seen or considered. Yet as a complication evolves, increasingly sophisticated skills are required. Table 1 suggests different skill levels that might be required; all cataract surgeons must be competent in Level 1 and Level 2 skills. The other core skills that should be learned include:

- techniques to convert from phaco to ECCE surgery
- alternative IOL implantation options
- suturing the eye
- anterior vitrectomy.

There are clear guidelines as to what should or should not be done and these rules are fundamental in setting objectives when managing a complication. Tissues in the eye are fragile, scarce and irreplaceable, with the exception of vitreous. Whereas capsule, iris and cornea must be conserved and handled with the greatest of care, the vitreous must always be removed and the anterior chamber left free of it at the end of the operation. Surgical repair should leave no tissue under tension, or compressed by a clumsily inserted IOL.

Table 1.1 Skills hierarchy for cataract surgery

Level 1	**Core skills for routine surgery**
	Wound construction
	Capsulorrhexis/capsulotomy
	Nucleus removal (phaco or expression)
	Cortical toilet
	IOL implantation
	Wound closure
Level 2	**Core skills for managing complications**
	Wound reconstruction for conversion to ECCE surgery
	ECCE skills including nuclear expression and completing the capsulotomy
	Suturing the wound
	Anterior vitrectomy
Level 3	**Advanced skills for managing complex problems**
	Retrieval of nuclear fragments or dislocated IOLs from the posterior segment
	Repositioning of decentered IOLs
	Scleral- or iris-fixation of posterior chamber IOLs
	IOL exchange or piggy-back lenses for incorrect power
	Refractive surgery

When struggling with a difficult case, remember the cardinal steps of the operation. Nothing beats sound technique, particularly when the going gets tough. Those who trained during the extracapsular cataract extraction (ECCE) era are fortunate to have learned the core skills that this operation required (e.g. cutting a section, suturing a wound or performing cortical toilet etc.). These skills helped their transition of technique to phacoemulsification and remain useful and can be called upon when a complication occurs. Nowadays, however, trainees pass directly to phaco without first learning the various skills of ECCE surgery and so are less well equipped when things go wrong. For this reason, we include a section on how to do a routine ECCE as well as a straightforward description of phacoemulsification by the technique of nuclear fractis.

Good preoperative decisions support good surgical outcomes. Anticipation and planning are necessary. Sometimes during the assessment process problems are noticed that could make an operation difficult, e.g. co-existing ocular pathology; lack of a special instrument; or if the available surgeon is inexperienced and the case difficult.

The value of good anaesthetic support cannot be stressed too highly. Remembering a difficult experience with a patient when their first eye was operated on, should suggest that a different approach, perhaps using a different anaesthetic technique, might be a safer way forward when the other eye is being considered. With hindsight, many complications will be seen to have been predictable at the time of listing or preoperative assessment. Some patients pose problems of cooperation during surgery, some eyes pose technical difficulties. If not appreciated preoperatively, either can cause serious problems during the operation. Preoperative examination should identify the routine from the risky case and allow you to prepare to match the operative technique to the problem. Anticipation of potential problems may allow obvious pitfalls to be avoided.

Similarly, because the skill or experience of surgeons vary, it is important to recognize that what may be difficult for one surgeon, may be better accomplished by another with a different skill base. Understanding one's limits is a mark of one's competence.

Every eye unit is experiencing pressure to increase the throughput of cataract patients. To cope with such large numbers, techniques close in style to production line methods are being used in some hospitals. The operative handling of patients is broken down into a series of steps, each extra layer of activity requiring more staff disrupting continuity of care and introducing opportunities for adverse events. Paramedical staff are given roles in patient management previously reserved for medical staff and in some developing countries nurses are trained to do extracapsular cataract surgery. Against this crescendo of activity it is important to reflect on the issue of patient safety and remember that it is a patient who suffers when a complication occurs. One must not try to blame the system or seek to hide a casualty in the large throughput. It is up to the surgeons, both senior and junior, to remember their crucial influence in the safe delivery of each and every operation. Preventing and managing complications depends not only on sound surgical techniques but also on the maintenance of good codes of practice and unimpeachable standards of sterility in the operating theatre. In the clinic, the appropriate listing and preoperative work-up of cases and careful postoperative management support good surgical outcomes. All these factors are necessary to avoid disasters and contain risk.

The surgeon should not only be able to recognize and respond to a complication, but should be able to reflect positively on those cases that go awry. By routinely doing this, surgeons learn how to avoid similar problems in the future, and perhaps gain insight into their real ability to respond when the going gets rough. Auditing of one's results is a formal exercise which focuses on outcomes and although it may reveal complications, it will fail to demonstrate 'near-misses' or adverse events which did not, but could have, caused mischief. Necessarily, the responsibility for continuing good practice requires a commitment to audit and the improvement of deficiencies if they occur, whether surgical, equipment, systems or judgement. Wrapped in the terminology of the present as 'clinical governance', there is corporate responsibility to improve and provide evidence of high standards of practice. This requires contributions from not only the surgeon and his or her team, juniors in training, nurses, professionals such as opticians and orthoptists, but also the senior management of the particular hospital. It is management's respon-

Worked Example: bilateral cataract surgery with complications

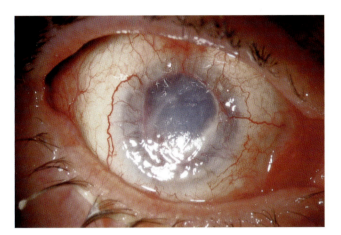

Fig. (a) Right eye with total corneal oedema

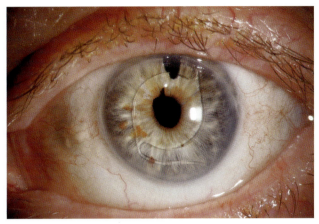

Fig. (b) Left eye showing ACIOL, D-shaped pupil indicating vitreous incarceration

A 67-year-old male underwent bilateral simultaneous ECCE cataract surgery. Right eye, post-capsular rupture with vitreous loss. AC IOL implanted. Left eye, operation proceeded with capsule rupture and again vitreous loss. AC IOL inserted.

Four years later referred for second opinion. C/o: Pain, poor vision. Findings: Right eye: PL, pseudophakic bullous keratopathy, soft eye. Left: 6/9, note D-shaped pupil indicating vitreous incarcerated in the section and around the IOL.

Advice: Right eye, poor prognosis even with corneal graft, removal IOL, anterior vitrectomy. Left eye, observe; risk of later retinal detachment.

Outcome: Right eye becomes phthisical. Patient dies 6 months later.

Critique: Adequate anterior vitrectomy essential at primary operation; symmetrical complication may be expected, and no surprises when capsular rupture occurred at the second operation.

Lesson: If complication occurs in first eye, delay surgery to fellow eye until the outcome from first operation is clear.

sibility to see that your reasonable needs of equipment, staffing and instrumentation are in place for you to discharge your duties properly and safely.

When things have gone wrong the eternally delicate issue of telling and talking to patients remains and is unavoidable. It is hoped that by honestly presenting and clearly discussing any problem with patients, they and their relatives can be brought 'on-side' and become involved in dealing with the problem and achieving the visual goals set prior to the operation. The final chapter deals straightforwardly with this, but also underlines the principles of good practice that will be your best ally if the unthinkable happens and you end up on the receiving end of litigation.

Part One

Routine Cataract Surgery

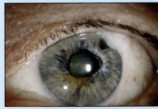

1 Preoperative assessment

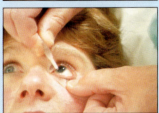

2 Anaesthetic considerations

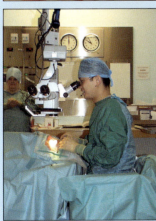

3 Standard surgical techniques: phacoemulsification and extracapsular cataract surgery

Chapter 1

Preoperative assessment

INTRODUCTION

The reported good outcomes from cataract surgery may blind outside observers to the risks or difficulties experienced during surgery. Awareness of risk is needed at every stage of the patient's care from the first examination until discharge after the operation.

Careful history-taking, accurate elucidation of relevant general and ophthalmic signs and wariness during surgery, supported by appropriate surgical experience sharpen this appreciation. Visual and functional difficulties must be noted and if signs of cataract are present, the patient may be listed for surgery. The notes should state the intended surgery, lens power and other details, such as which anaesthetic method is to be used, and whether the operation is required as a day case or through admission to the ward. If new factors come to light there will be opportunities to change the surgical plan.

CLINIC VISIT

A patient has been referred to you for consideration of cataract surgery. A clinic consultation should establish whether lens opacities play a major role in the patient's symptoms and what potential systemic and ophthalmological problems may occur that might complicate surgery.

History

The first contact with a patient is very important. For many, the fear of blindness may be their strongest emotion. Even if this is the tenth time in this clinic you have had to go through a similar consultation, it is the first and only time for this particular patient. Each person should be treated individually and not as though they have been plucked from a conveyor belt.

Why is the patient is sitting in your consulting room? They may have been referred by a well-meaning optometrist or general practitioner but they themselves are unaware of any difficulties. More commonly, however, the patient will have visual symptoms. These may be reduced visual acuity, glare from artificial or natural light or monocular diplopia. Although all cataracts can produce symptoms, nuclear cataracts tend to reduce vision, posterior subcapsular cataracts will affect vision and lead to glare whereas cortical opacities will scatter light causing glare and monocular diplopia.

Are you sure that it is a cataract that is causing the patient's symptoms? There may be co-existing ocular pathology; macular degeneration and glaucoma are also age-related diseases. Cataracts can co-exist with diabetic maculopathy. Problems with reading or metamorphopsia can suggest that despite the presence of nuclear sclerosis, the patient's principal problem is macular and not lenticular.

What does the reduced or compromised vision stop the patient from doing? For instance, if an elderly woman can read, knit, watch television and care for herself with visions of 6/12, the risks of surgery may outweigh the potential benefits. If a professional golfer, with a vision of 6/9, has problems with glare, it may be worth the risk to remove the cataracts.

Is there anything in the past ocular history that might lead to more complicated surgery? For instance, if the patient has suffered blunt ocular trauma, the lens may be unstable; previous uveitis or the use of pilocarpine drops may prevent the pupil from dilating fully; a patient may have had previous ocular surgery, e.g. trabeculectomy, retinal detachment surgery or a vitrectomy (posterior subcapsular opacities invariably follow vitreous/gas exchanges).

What systemic problems does the patient suffer from and which could affect safe surgery? For instance, the patient may be on warfarin for heart or large vessel disease; poorly controlled hypertension can increase the risk of a suprachoroidal haemorrhage and untreated is a relative contraindication to certain anaesthetic techniques.

Congestive heart failure, chronic obstructive airways disease, head tremor, perseveration of the blink reflex in Parkinson's and spinal kyphosis or arthritis may make it impossible for the patient to lie flat or still. Some systemic disorders may lead to problems with the anaesthetic. These latter issues will be covered in the next chapter.

Ophthalmic examination

VISION

Visual acuity should be measured both with and without correction and with a pin-hole if indicated. Glare can be simulated by shining a light from the side, while the patient is reading the chart. Dense or mature cataracts cause very poor vision and restrict the view of the posterior segment. Check that the patient does not have a relative afferent pupillary defect; this would suggest a major retinal or neurological problem. The ability to project light accurately is also a helpful way of assessing retinal function. If there is a dense lens opacity, a clear ultrasound B-scan is essential to reassure you that there are no gross problems behind the lens. Remember that neurological disease can also cause reduced vision and if the lens opacities are not significant, check the patient's colour vision and visual fields to exclude chiasmal compression or a homonymous hemianopia.

OCULAR MOVEMENTS

A full orthoptic examination is rarely required but a history of a squint should warn about the possibility of postoperative diplopia, or amblyopia causing a poor visual result. If a squint is noted it should be carefully documented; it may have developed as a consequence of the reduced vision (i.e. decompensation of a previous phoria) or it may have been present since childhood. Recent onset strabismus has a higher risk of causing postoperative diplopia and the patient should be warned accordingly.

SLIT-LAMP

The ocular examination should be systematic, moving from front to back, i.e. periorbita, lids, conjunctiva, cornea, anterior chamber, IOP, lens, vitreous, optic nerve and retina. Abnormal signs in each of the anatomical areas can be associated with a particular set of potential complications (see Table 1.1). It is as important to document negative and positive findings. It demonstrates thoroughness and will ensure you examine the eye carefully and fully.

If any problems are found that may affect the outcome of surgery, you should initiate treatment, e.g. glaucoma, blepharitis or uveitis. Blepharitis should be treated with a programme of lid hygiene and topical antibiotics, but if severe, surgery should be postponed. Active uveitis must be controlled and the eye should have been 'quiet' for at least 3 months before operating; a pulse of intravenous methyl prednisolone can be given peroperatively to further minimize the chance of a flare-up.

If co-existing ocular pathology is likely to reduce the visual gain, a guarded prognosis must be given to the patient, e.g. glaucoma and macular degeneration.

Look carefully at the lens. Learn to estimate the hardness of the lens and anticipate the potential difficulties you will encounter. Look at its different layers and colour, and estimate the size of the nucleus. Brunescent lenses are

Table 1.1 A directed preoperative examination

Structure	Sign	Potential surgical complication
Lids	inflamed, crusts	endophthalmitis
Conjunctiva	inflamed, discharge	endophthalmitis
Cornea	scar in visual axis	poor perop. visibility
	thickening, haze, guttata	corneal decompensation
	keratic precipitates	postop. inflammation
Anterior chamber	shallow	little surgical room
	cells/flare	postop. inflammation
IOP (and blood pressure)	raised	suprachoroidal haemorrhage
Pupil margin	pseudoexfoliation	zonular rupture
Iris	damaged/synechiae	postop. inflammation
	synechiae	small pupil
Lens	brunescent cataract	corneal decompensation
		prolonged surgery
		zonular rupture
	white/mature cataract	difficult capsulorrhexis
	capsular scar	hole in posterior capsule
Peripheral retina	lattice degeneration	retinal detachment
Other eye	previous complication	similar problem may occur

usually very hard with large nuclei, and may require more manipulation and phaco energy for its removal than another lens of lighter colour. Consider whether the case would be better dealt with using a chopping technique. They are not ideal cases for the tyro phaco surgeon. In these cases, the apparent disadvantages of ECCE may be offset if the surgeon is competent at ECCE and where speed and ease of removal are important.

It is useful, at least initially, when examining the lens to attempt to record the lens morphology pictorially (Fig. 1.1). This simple grading system invites a thoughtful approach to the examination of the lens and provides a useful, at-a-glance *aide-mémoire* which will be useful in the operating room.

Identify and record active or theoretically problematic conditions which may be made worse by surgery (think too, about ploys that may moderate adverse effects):

(a) Diabetic maculopathy may deteriorate; early laser may be required.

(b) Retinitis pigmentosa; cystoid macular oedema frequently develops: treat with acetazolamide.

(c) Steroid-responder; use minimal postoperative steroids to avoid raised intraocular pressure.

(d) Previous uveitis; possibility of aggressive postoperative inflammation: give IV methyl prednisolone on induction of anaesthesia.

(e) Corneal endothelial degenerations (e.g. Fuch's endothelial dystrophy); postoperative corneal oedema possible. Be prepared to use a viscoelastic such as Viscoat or Healonid 5 to help protect the endothelium. Combined corneal graft and cataract operation may be indicated. Special care is required; the surgery should be performed by a more experienced surgeon.

The history and examination should be well documented and supported by diagrams or drawings where appropri-

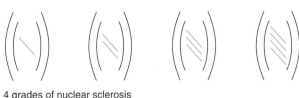

4 grades of nuclear sclerosis
Use the cross hatching to indicate hardness

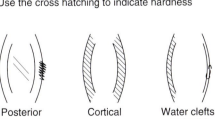

| Posterior subcapsular lens opacities | Cortical lens opacities | Water clefts and mild nuclear sclerosis | Combine cortical and nuclear sclerosis |

Fig. 1.1 Drawing of lenses

ate. It should be useful and relevant to that patient and to you in their surgical care and recovery. The cardinal findings should be clear and easily found.

Patient information

To be given the diagnosis of 'cataracts' can be a body blow, especially to a patient who may be struggling with other health issues. By explaining the diagnosis and the likely outcomes of surgery, you will reassure the patient. Any special risks of surgery should be identified as well as the measures needed to contain them. It is the surgeon's duty to mould the patient's expectations to fit the spectrum of likely outcomes and a realistic prognosis should be offered. Draw patients into the decision-making process encouraging them to be partners in the care being offered. This shared understanding of potential problems helps both the surgeon and the patient accept a less favourable outcome. If the patient is happy to continue, then list them for surgery.

Listing for surgery

Having assessed the patient, discussed their problems and established the need for surgery, the surgeon must tell the patient what is planned in plain English or through an interpreter. A concise record of what is to be done should now be written. If the examining doctor is junior, the intention to list should be discussed with the surgeon in charge. This gives the consultant an opportunity to check unusual findings and to agree to planned treatment. Record, if relevant, any potential complexities of the case and suggest the level of surgeon who should do the surgery, e.g. consultant only. It is customary to operate on the eye with the worst vision first, provided of course that both eyes have the same visual potential.

These clinic notes will remind you of any special issues and strategies to be followed when the patient arrives for surgery. This is crucial when the gap between surgery and listing is prolonged, and especially if the next, preop. examination is to be by a nurse or junior doctor.

A decision should also be made as to the type of anaesthesia that is most appropriate (see Chapter 2). Any preoperative treatment required should be started.

Although some surgeons feel that bilateral simultaneous surgery can be routinely offered, in the authors' experience, there are relatively few indications for this approach. A likely scenario would be a very elderly patient living alone, presenting with dense bilateral cataracts, and who had a relative who was only able to visit for a short or single visit to support the patient through the perioperative period.

Remembering that bilateral peribulbar and retrobulbar anaesthesia may use volumes of local anaesthetic which approach toxic levels, a case can be made to remove both cataracts using a general anaesthetic. Ask the anaesthetist about the patient's fitness. Alternatively, surgery under topical anaesthesia is another option.

An overriding rule when offering such surgery is to state clearly that the second eye will only be done if the operation on the first eye was uncomplicated (see the Worked Example in the Introduction). A complication of the first operation may be repeated in the second eye. The potential risk of bilateral complications such as endophthalmitis is extremely small but such advice must be specifically incorporated into any preoperative counselling. Particular care is also needed to treat each operation as entirely separate, using different instruments, fluids and solutions with different batch numbers to ensure that contamination does not occur.

Assessment of technical difficulty

Drawing on all the facts garnered at the examination, learn to assess the technical difficulty each eye poses.

Brown lenses in elderly patients tend to be the hardest and consequently the most challenging. Other co-existing ocular pathology and problems with the patient's general health may convert a technically 'easy' cataract operation into very challenging surgery. Boxes 1.1–1.3 indicate a suggested method for grading lenses and how such a classification may help to indicate the level of surgeon that should undertake the procedure.

'Standard risk' cases are most appropriate for training purposes; these are the most suitable for inexperienced trainees under supervision or those working independently for the first time. Intermediate risk cases can be operated on by more experienced surgeons or by senior trainees under supervision. Only those with sufficient experience and expertise, e.g. consultants, experienced trainees or fellows under supervision, should undertake the high risk cases.

By making a habit of estimating the clinical difficulty you will learn to anticipate problems and plan for appropriate instrumentation and time. Cases should be allocated on the basis of the experience and competence required for their safe completion. Realistic expectations of outcomes and problems can then be presented to the patient.

Box 1.1 Standard risk surgery

EYE

- Nuclear sclerotic cataract
- Lamellar cataract

PATIENT

- Patient able to lie flat and still
- First eye, or second eye after successful first eye surgery

Box 1.2 Intermediate risk surgery

EYE

- Cataract in a young patient
- Corneal guttata, moderate, marked
- Corneal opacity, focal or diffuse
- Posterior synechiae/history of uveitis
- Brunescent cataract
- Small pupil
- White, mature cataract
- Previous trauma
- Previous glaucoma surgery
- Previous corneal graft
- Previous vitreo-retinal surgery
- Pseudoexfoliation syndrome
- High myopes/nanophthalmia

PATIENT PROBLEMS

- Only eye/fellow eye amblyopic
- Previous complicated cataract surgery
- Systemic problems affecting operating position (i.e speed of surgery is important) – kyphosis
- Orthopnoea, high anxiety

Box 1.3 High risk surgery

EYE

- Combinations of those listed under increased risk
- Unstable lens (developmental or post-traumatic)
- Pseudoexfoliation
- Previous perforating injury suspected of involving the posterior capsule
- Emergency surgery on an inflamed eye, e.g. phacomorphic glaucoma

PATIENT

- Concurrent ocular condition affecting visual prognosis especially in the younger patient, e.g. retinitis pigmentosa, aniridia
- Poor general health, e.g. COAD, CCF, Parkinson's disease
- Previous anaesthetic problems, major cardiovascular disease
- Social problems – likely poor compliance with drops postop., dementia

COMBINATIONS OF ALL THE ABOVE

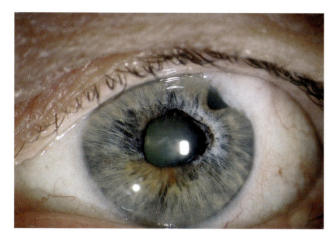

Fig. 1.2 Brunescent cataract

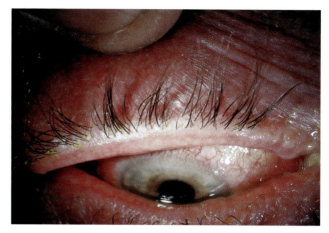

Fig. 1.5 Blepharitis

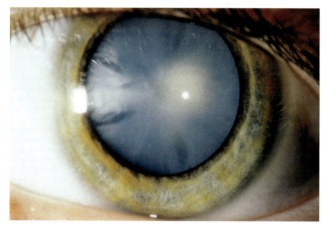

Fig. 1.3 Mature cataract

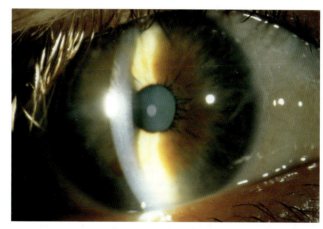

Fig. 1.6 Fuch's endothelial dystrophy

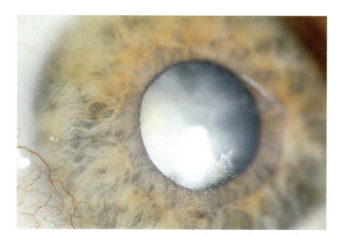

Fig. 1.4 Phacomorphic glaucoma

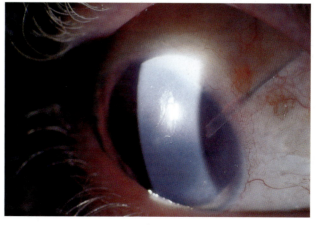

Fig. 1.7 Cataract with seton in place

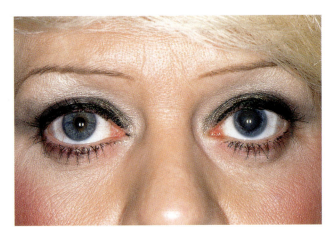

Fig. 1.8 Fuch's heterochromic iridocyclitis

PREOPERATIVE VISIT/ ASSESSMENT

Sometimes because of waiting lists and patterns of working, patients may wait many months between the initial clinic visit and their surgery. The clinical picture might change and it is important to review the patient nearer the time of operation. A quick run-through of the important issues should be done.

Biometry

Whether completed during the first consultation or at a separate preoperative visit, the power and lens style will need to be assessed. This requires the following information:

(a) corrected and uncorrected vision in both eyes
(b) knowledge of earliest and recent refraction (focimetry or optician's prescription)
(c) keratometry
(d) measurement of axial length.

Biometry must always be done on *both* eyes – this is important and provides an immediate internal control on the readings. In most patients the axial lengths and keratometry findings should be similar for the two eyes. Any asymmetry in the readings must be questioned and the readings repeated until you are sure of their accuracy. If there is a history of anisometropia, the axial length and IOL power should reflect this difference, e.g. if the axial lengths are dissimilar in a myopic patient, the eye with the longer axial length should have been the more myopic. Similarly, the calculated IOL power should be different by approximately the same difference in power of the patient's spectacles.

Use the recommended A constant for the lens in your calculation, but back-check by auditing the refractive outcomes, that the constant chosen gives repeatable and accurate results in the range that you want. The A constant can be varied if there is a trend to myopic or hypermetropic outcomes. If your unit constantly produces outcomes that are hypermetropic, increase the A constant by 0.50, e.g. an A constant of 118.5 could be increased to 119.0 if the results were trending to plus (+) 1.00; check and increase again if they are improved but still too long-sighted. (Do not do this without checking with your colleagues! Their refractive results may be uniformly better than yours.)

Remember that if the indicated lens powers for the two eyes are very different, the difference should be consistent with the preoperative spectacle refraction. If the readings seem bizarre, you should re-check the readings and repeat the measurements until you are satisfied with their accuracy.

Some reasons for experiencing difficulty in carrying out biometry are listed in Box 1.4.

> **Box 1.4** Reasons for difficulty in doing biometry
>
> ▶ Poor tear film
> ▶ Recent applanation
> ▶ Uncooperative patient (e.g. child)
> ▶ Previous corneal graft or other surface irregularities
> ▶ Ptosis
> ▶ Squint

Both long and short eyes need special programmes and calculations to ensure biometric accuracy. For long eyes with axial lengths greater than 26 mm, the SRK Theoretic formula is said to be more accurate. Similarly for short eyes, the Hoffer calculation is recommended. You should also remember that the unusual power lenses that may be needed for these unusual eyes may not be routinely available and may need to be specifically ordered.

Biometry will identify patients with exceptional axial lengths and for whom it may be safer to use a general anaesthetic. It is our routine to offer general anaesthesia to our highly myopic patients as they may present a greater risk for perforation with peribulbar anaesthesia (see Chapter 2).

The surgeon remains responsible for ensuring that the correct IOL is chosen and used, even though biometry is increasingly frequently done by non-medical personnel.

The surgical plan

A surgical plan should be drawn up and adhered to. This means recording which eye is to be operated on, the IOL power and style, the chosen anaesthetic and the selected surgeon. This information should be entered into the medical notes and be included on the published operating list.

THE DAY OF SURGERY

Patients should be welcomed onto the ward and when they come to the operating theatre. Introductions should be made at the bed-side rather than in the operating room when the patient is lying flat on the table. Running through a simple checklist (Box 1.5) will avoid mistakes and will reaffirm the agreed surgical plan.

Preoperative preparation

The preoperative preparation of the eye sets the scene for safe surgery. Ensure that the dilating drops are correctly prescribed on the drug chart. Maximal pupillary dilation should be obtained and a suggested regimen is presented in Box 1.6.

In the operating theatre

Before starting to operate, the surgeon must be sure that the patient has been correctly identified, that the consent form is signed and that the operation is the correct procedure on the intended side. These systems of checking are fundamental to good practice. If the systems are ignored and a problem occurs, then the matter will be legally indefensible. The issues surrounding obtaining consent will be covered in a later chapter.

Box 1.5 Surgeon's preoperative check-list

▶ Check all the records and remind yourself of the problems identified at the pre-assessment visit, e.g. the presence of pseudoexfoliation or unusual biometry
▶ Check which eye is to be operated on. Does this agree with the consent form and the notes (*some surgeons prefer to mark the forehead over the eye*)
▶ Check, again, the biometry print-out and the IOL chosen. Is it consistent with what you would expect for the patient's preoperative refraction?
▶ Check the chosen lens power and style
▶ Check that the preoperative medication has been prescribed and that the drops have been written for the correct side
▶ Check that the patient is whom you think he/she should be! Patients with the same name can sometimes cause confusion

---

Box 1.6 Preoperative regimen to dilate pupil

PREOP. DROPS

▶ Instil drops 4× in the hour before surgery:
▶ G. cyclopentolate 1%
▶ G. phenylephrine 2.5% or 10%
▶ (G. voltarol is also used by some surgeons)
▶ Prophylactic antibiotic: G. chloramphenicol

Chapter 2

Anaesthetic considerations

INTRODUCTION

Each surgical team will have their own preferred anaesthetic requirements for their surgical routine. With the anaesthetist, they will agree on the appropriate techniques to be used, and although a specific technique can be favoured, there are occasions when a choice needs to be made from the range of topical anaesthesia through to general anaesthesia, for a particular patient. Discussion is important in choosing the appropriate technique, as the surgeon and anaesthetist will look at the patient from different aspects, and a compromise, taking into account the wishes of the patient, is appropriate.

ROLE OF THE ANAESTHETIST

The role of the anaesthetist varies from surgical team to surgical team and the case-mix in their workload. Most importantly, good working relationships with anaesthetists will ensure the best and safest journey by the patient through the operative experience. Good anaesthetic input will help avoid surgical difficulties and prevent patient discomfort.

You should encourage the anaesthetist's involvement in patient support during the perioperative phase, recruiting their participation to act as the physician to the surgical team, and modifying medical treatment to improve the patient's condition (some even advocate that anaesthetists should be retitled as 'perioperative physicians'!). During surgery they will then be available to provide any of several anaesthetic choices to permit safe and comfortable surgery for patient and surgeon alike, e.g. by performing the local anaesthetic block or giving a general anaesthetic.

The anaesthetist's involvement may be limited, for instance when a surgical team wishes to perform the local anaesthetics themselves; here, the anaesthetist's role may be to provide intravenous access, and supervise monitoring of the patient, being available to help if problems occur.

PREOPERATIVE ANAESTHETIC ASSESSMENT

This should be arranged on the basis of a pre-agreed protocol. Problems requiring anaesthetic advice may include patients for either local or general anaesthesia with medical problems, especially if they suffer with angina, orthopnoea, or dyspnoea on minor exertion. In that changes in treatment may take several weeks to become effective, early consultation is important so that appropriate plans can be made.

The general fitness of a patient is now often expressed in terms of the ASA status. This refers to the American Society of Anesthesiologists Physical Status Scale, which correlates with the risk of anaesthesia and surgery.

- Class I   A normally healthy individual
- Class II   A patient with mild systemic disease
- Class III   A patient with severe systemic disease that is not incapacitating
- Class IV   A patient with incapacitating systemic disease that is a constant threat to life
- Class V   A moribund patient who is not expected to survive 24 hours with or without operation

The anaesthetist's involvement is particularly relevant in ASA III and IV patients who may have difficulties even with local anaesthesia, often due to an inability to lie flat.

Most medication is now continued up to the time of surgery, but some do interact with general anaesthetic agents: this is the province of the anaesthetist, but simple problems to be avoided include hypokalaemia with diuretics (tendency to arrhythmias), use of monoamine oxidase inhibitors (hypertensive reactions with some narcotic analgesics), significant anaemia (below 10 g/dl) and major anticoagulation. These can all be identified at preliminary assessment.

Anticoagulation

Anticoagulation is a debatable problem, as basic anaesthetic teaching is that local anaesthetic blocks are not performed in patients taking these agents, while the ophthalmic literature contains contrasting opinions. The risk of significant bleeding with an INR of 2 is acceptable, so it is reasonable to request that anticoagulants are reduced to obtain this level of anticoagulation. At this level, surgery and local anaesthetic blocks can be performed with less risk.

TECHNIQUES OF ANAESTHESIA

Local anaesthesia

Every technique has its enthusiasts, but none is without its own benefits and risks.

There are three main types of local anaesthesia used during eye surgery, topical, sub-Tenon's and peribulbar injection of local anaesthetic; a fourth technique, retrobulbar, is now used less frequently because of the higher incidence of complications.

TOPICAL

Here only superficial anaesthesia is provided initially, with intracameral injection or infusion of dilute local anaesthetic providing anaesthesia for deeper structures. Topical anaesthesia can be provided with proxymetacaine (minimal stinging), benoxinate (stings initially, fairly effective) or amethocaine (stings initially, effective, but corneal epithelial clouding may occur). Prior administration of dilute solutions of any of these agents, at approximately one-tenth strength, minimizes any discomfort; the use of lignocaine gel is an alternative. For some patients this degree of analgesia is sufficient for them to cope quite happily with their cataract operation.

Additional analgesia can be provided by intracameral injection of local anaesthetic using preservative-free 1% lignocaine.

A small subconjunctival injection of 2% lignocaine may be performed superiorly to facilitate insertion of a superior rectus stay suture.

With these combined techniques, adequate analgesia is common, but free movement persists, which may be unacceptable in some situations and especially for the learner surgeon. The patient may experience a sensation of pressure during intraocular manipulations, and should be warned of this in advance.

RETROBULBAR BLOCK

This has been widely used for many years, and results in akinesia and anaesthesia of the structures of the eye. A transcutaneous approach, after preliminary infiltration, is used to pass a 1.25 inch 25G or smaller needle, entering just above the infra-orbital rim at the junction between the middle and outer thirds of the eye. The needle is passed parallel to the axis of the globe until the point is judged to be beyond the equator of the globe, when the needle angle is adjusted so that it passes medially and up, into the muscle cone behind the globe. Asking the patient to move the eye away from the primary position as the needle is passed (the classical teaching is to tell the patient to 'look upwards and inwards') brings the optic nerve forwards and increases the risk of it being impaled. Inject about 3 ml of adrenaline-free local anaesthetic (inject slowly to avoid discomfort).

An oculopression device such as a 'super Pinkie' or 'Honan balloon' is then applied for 10 min to produce softening of the eye. The balloon is set to a pressure of approximately 30 mmHg. The lids should be closed with tape and the eye padded with gauze beneath the device. Traditionally a block of the facial nerve to paralyse the orbicularis oculi is also given.

This block has the risks of globe perforation, retrobulbar haemorrhage, intravascular injection, intraneural injection and central spread of local anaesthetic: these are rare but potentially devastating.

SUB-TENON'S BLOCK

This can be achieved after topical anaesthesia by passing an appropriate blunt tipped cannula through a conjunctival incision 5 mm from the limbus, generally in the inferior nasal area, after blunt dissection to expose the sclera under Tenon's capsule. One ml of adrenaline-free anaesthetic solution is injected beyond the equator of the globe, then after further advance, up to 3 ml is injected. Lignocaine 2% is suitable, but for a more prolonged block, can be mixed with bupivacaine 0.5%. Good analgesia, but with a varying degree of akinesia, is obtained. Reported complications are minimal.

PERIBULBAR BLOCK

The classic sites for two injections are inferotemporal, and medial to the supra-orbital notch, but this latter site is now less favoured, and many prefer a site medial to the caruncle (see Fig. 2.4). Satisfactory blocks can be obtained with injection at only one site, but better akinesia is achieved when two sites are used. Transcutaneous injections after preliminary infiltration can be used, but others prefer transconjunctival injections after topical anaesthesia is achieved.

Topical anaesthesia is provided by administration of dilute, then full-strength benoxinate until the patient has no sensation when further drops are administered (see Fig. 2.1).

The local anaesthetic solutions used for injection vary, but a popular mixture is

5 ml 2% lignocaine with 1:200 000 adrenaline
+
5 ml 0.75% bupivacaine
+
hyaluronidase 500–1500 i.u.

Some omit adrenaline, while others add freshly prepared dilute adrenaline. Postoperative analgesia for about 4 hours is likely.

Use of 2% prilocaine, with or without 0.75% bupivacaine, is possible, but the stronger preparations of prilocaine are licensed for dental use only: they have been used by some workers, but the complications encountered have drawn attention to the restrictions of the product licence. The recently introduced agents ropivacaine (Naropin) and levo-bupivacaine (Chirocaine) have their advocates: they have lower systemic toxicity, especially in terms of cardiac effects, but their use is not yet widespread. Blocks performed with 0.75% bupivacaine alone may result in diplopia the next day.

A 1 inch (25 mm) needle of 25G or smaller is used, and passed to just beyond the equator of the globe, parallel to the axis of the globe. The needle is passed with the eye in the primary position (see Figs 2.3 and 2.4), but before injecting the patient should be asked to move the eye to show that the ocular tissues are clear of the needle. Inject 4–6 ml of local anaesthetic solution. After gentle pressure applied to the orbit for about 30 seconds, a similar injection at the second site can be given (Figs 2.5 and 2.6).

An alternative approach is to apply an oculopression device for 10 min; if using a Honan's balloon the pressure is generally set to 30 mmHg (see Fig. 2.8). Then assess whether a second injection is required. The lids should be closed with tape (Fig. 2.7) and the eye padded with gauze beneath the device. Orbicularis paresis is generally obtained by spread of the anaesthetic solution to the terminal branches of the facial nerve. If after adequate time has elapsed for the block to become established, there is still troublesome movement persisting, top-up injections can be given at a site relevant for block of the appropriate nerve, but remembering the problem of local anaesthetic toxicity.

Figs 2.1–2.12 show the various steps in preparing a patient for theatre with a peribulbar block.

There is often some discomfort during the injection of the large volumes used, and various techniques have been used to reduce this. These include warming the solution to 37°C (Fig. 2.2) (also affects pKa and hence speeds onset), prior injection of large volumes of dilute solutions (e.g. 1 ml of local diluted in 9 ml of warmed normal saline), and infiltration of small volumes of dilute solutions at the injection sites. The variety of techniques used perhaps indicates that a perfect answer to the problem of pain on injection has yet to be found.

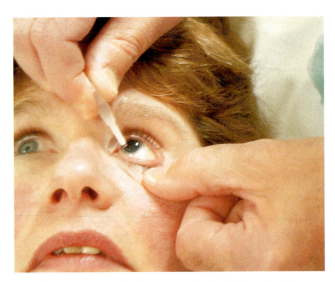

Fig. 2.1 Local anaesthetic drops are applied until the patient is unaware of further drops being instilled

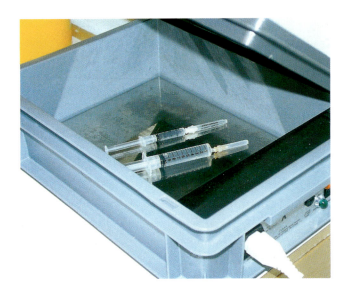

Fig. 2.2 The solutions of local anaesthetic are first placed in a warming cabinet

Peribulbar local anaesthesia still has the risk of globe perforation, but the other risks are reduced, as the needle does not enter the muscle cone. Some inject proximal to the equator of the globe, but many inject just distal to the equator. Larger volumes (up to 10 ml) are used, and local anaesthetic toxicity can be a problem in the frail patient, especially if large volumes (including top-up injections) of concentrated solutions are used (Table 2.1).

The concept of local anaesthetic toxicity is complicated because most cases are probably due to accidental intravascular injection. In general, the site of injection alters the rate of absorption and thus the eventual local anaesthetic

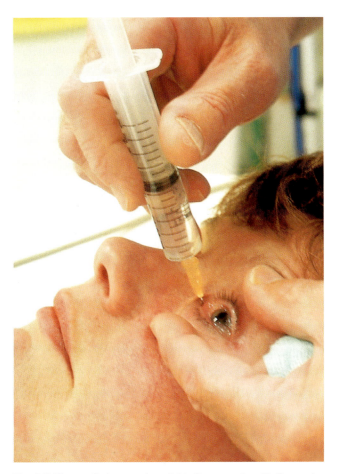

Fig. 2.3 The needle is passed medial to the caruncle, with the eye in the primary position

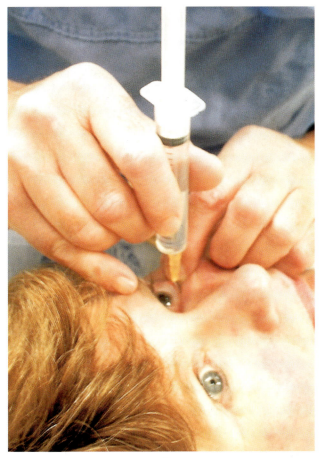

Fig. 2.5 Injection at a second site, via the conjunctiva inferolaterally

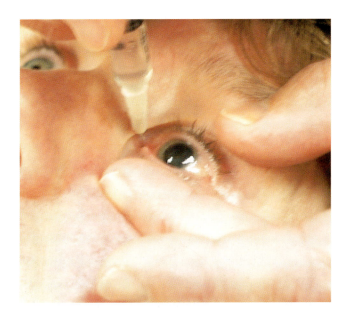

Fig. 2.4 Local anaesthetic is injected only after checking to see that the eye can move freely

Table 2.1 Maximum doses of local anaesthetic agents

Agent	Maximum dose		
	mg	70 kg	max. volume
Lignocaine plain	3 mg/kg	c.200 mg	10 ml 2%
Lignocaine with 1 in 200 000 adrenaline	7 mg/kg	c.500 mg	25 ml 2%
Bupivacaine	2 mg/kg	c.150 mg	20 ml 0.75%
Prilocaine	6 mg/kg	c.400 mg	20 ml 2%

blood levels. Adrenaline results in a lower maximum blood level, but its effects vary with the local anaesthetic agent used.

Maximum recommended doses have been published, and they are unlikely to be exceeded with even high volume blocks for ophthalmic anaesthesia, but these maximum doses should probably be reduced in the more frail, elderly population having ophthalmic anaesthesia.

The choice of technique needs to be based upon the needs of the surgeon, but with the increasing use of pha-

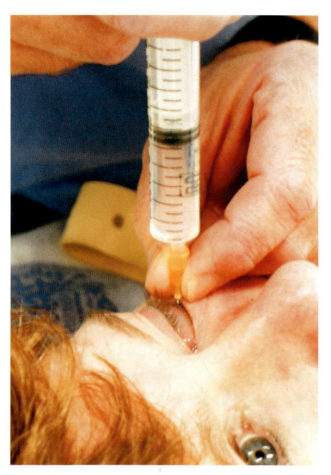

Fig. 2.6 Note chemosis developing as the extra injection is given

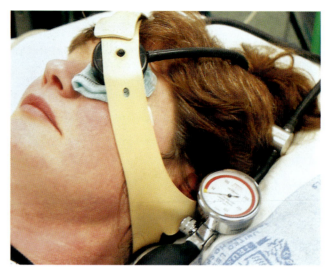

Fig. 2.8 A Honan's bulb is applied with the pressure set on 30 mmHg

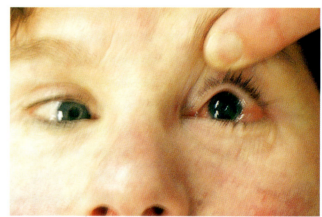

Fig. 2.9 This eye is both numb and unable to move

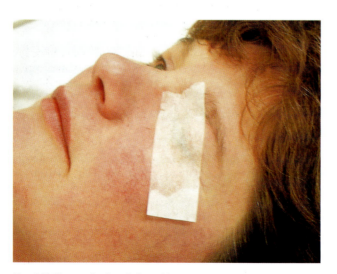

Fig. 2.7 The eye is closed shut with tape and covered with gauze

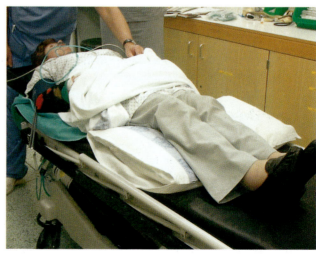

Fig. 2.10 A pillow is placed behind the patient's knees, improving their comfort

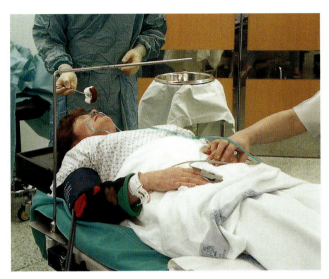

Fig. 2.11 In the theatre, the patient's hand is held, and extra oxygen is supplied with nasal cannulae

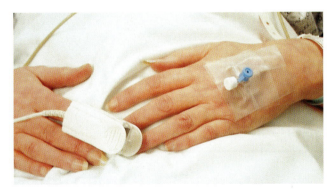

Fig. 2.12 Monitoring with an oxygen pulsimeter, and IV access is maintained via an indwelling intravenous cannula

coemulsification, topical, intracameral and sub-Tenon's methods are likely to prevail. Certainly the highly myopic eye in which there is a greater likelihood of a staphyloma being present is unsuitable for retrobulbar and most peri-bulbar techniques.

Patient comfort

With any local anaesthetic technique it is important that attention is given to the comfort of the patient. The patient should be kept warm (operating theatres are often cool for the comfort of the active well clothed workers) and judicious padding of the table may be required. A pillow under the knees reduces greatly the strain on the back from lying flat (see Fig. 2.10). It may be a great comfort to the patient to hold the hand of a staff member during the operation, and to be able to gain their attention by hand squeezing if there is a problem (see Fig. 2.11). Draping may restrict airflow to

the patient, who may feel a degree of claustrophobia. The drapes should be positioned to minimize this, and often oxygen or air can be given at low flow rates to the patient through nasal cannulae, or at higher flow rates from an anaesthetic circuit positioned loosely under the drapes. (Anaesthetic agents have accidentally been given in this way with anticipated effects on the patient.)

Patient monitoring

Minimal monitoring standards require the use of ECG monitoring, pulse oximetry and blood pressure measurement (see Fig. 2.12). However, it is disturbing to the patient to have automatic BP machines inflating and deflating during the operation; blood pressure should be checked both before performing a local anaesthetic block and if problems arise.

If pulse oximetry reveals hypoxia (less than 90% saturation), check the patient's condition (ask them how they are), look for a cause and treat appropriately: extra oxygen may be needed or oxygenation improved by attention to the airway.

PROBLEMS WITH LOCAL ANAESTHESIA

These are described more fully in Hamilton's chapter on 'Complications of ophthalmic regional anaesthesia' in Finucane's book. (See further reading list at the end of the chapter.)

1   Inadequate blocks: if a modest amount of movement persists, no further treatment may be needed, but if there is pain, extra local anaesthesia should be given, topically or by injection to obtain relief. Intravenous sedation is not the answer, and is likely to result in a restless and confused patient.

2   Retrobulbar haematoma: this can be arterial or venous in origin and may need urgent decompression. It is more likely with an intraconal than an extraconal injection (see Worked Example 2.1).

3   Brain stem anaesthesia: here there is direct spread from the orbit to the brain along the optic nerve, and it is rapid in onset, within a few minutes of the injection of the local anaesthetic. Symptoms range from confusion to respiratory arrest: treatment consists of postponing surgery, and extends from reassurance to full cardiorespiratory support. Problems should be suspected if there is confusion or loss of consciousness; shivering, nausea or vomiting; spread of the block to the other eye; difficulty in swallowing; respiratory depression and cardiovascular collapse. Do not hesitate to request immediate anaesthetic support as the condition may progress.

Worked Example 2.1

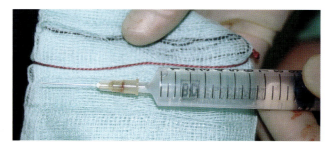

Fig. (a)

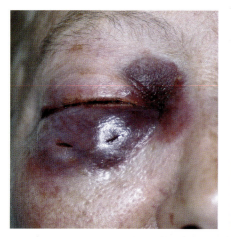

Fig. (b)

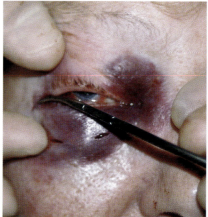

Fig. (c)

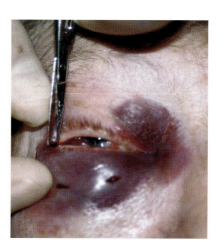

Fig. (d)

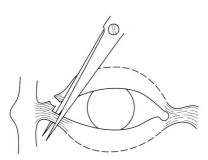

Fig. (e)

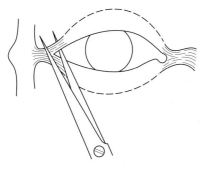

Fig. (f)

A healthy 73-year-old woman was brought into the anaesthetic room for peribulbar block. At the time of the first injection, the plunger of the syringe was gently withdrawn and bright red blood was aspirated (Fig. a). Immediately, this was followed by sudden and increasing proptosis and bruising of the lower lid which extended medially and superiorly. The orbit became very tense and the patient complained of pain and loss of sight. Note: no local had yet been injected.

Two stabs with a Bard–Parker number 15 blade through the orbital septum failed to release any haematoma (Fig. b). A lateral cantholysis was then carried out – initially the inferior and then the superior canthal tendons were cut with sharp-pointed scissors (Figs c and d) to decompress the orbit. There was immediate reduction in the orbital tension and a quick return of vision. These procedures are diagrammatically represented in Figs (e) and (f).

The eye was padded and the patient returned to the ward. She was checked 2 hours later and then discharged home. She was readmitted 6 weeks later and underwent uneventful cataract surgery under general anaesthetic.

4 Globe trauma: the real incidence of this problem is unknown as many cases are not reported, and the most minor cases may not be diagnosed. More than 50% of cases of globe trauma are undetected when they occur, but the problem should be suspected if the passage of the needle causes significant pain or there is resistance felt; intraocular injection of local anaesthetic is also very painful. After passage of the needle, the patient can be asked to look laterally: if globe movement is restricted, then penetration is likely to have occurred. This possibility must be further investigated. The diagnosis should be suspected if the eye is surprisingly soft, if there is a poor red reflex, or evidence of vitreous haemorrhage. Treatment extends from laser photocoagulation or cryotherapy, to vitrectomy, to formal retinal detachment surgery. There are conflicting opinions in the literature about the advantages and disadvantages of blunt- and sharp-tipped needles, but the problem should be less with peribulbar, extraconal injections and avoiding the use of needles greater than 25 mm in length: with intraconal injection, rates for globe trauma of approximately 1:1000 have been reported.

5 Ocular ischaemia: this may occur not only as a result of retrobulbar haemorrhage, but also from the use of oculopression devices, especially if there is significant local arterial disease or glaucoma. Some argue that adrenaline in the local anaesthetic mixture may contribute to the problem.

6 Optic nerve damage: this is a possibility with intraconal injection from direct trauma or from local pressure effects upon the blood supply to the nerve itself if intraneural injection occurs.

7 Muscle damage: this can result from intramuscular injection, or from the myotoxicity of the higher concentrations of local anaesthetic.

8 Oculocardiac reflex: this can occur when surgery is undertaken in the presence of incomplete anaesthesia, when there is traction on the extraocular muscles. Another vagally mediated problem is the vaso-vagal episode sometimes seen in needle-phobics and those prone to fainting: it can even occur at the time of insertion of the intravenous cannula.

9 Overdosage of local anaesthetic: this is unlikely with the use of normal volumes used even for peribulbar block, but may occur with the accumulated total dosage if supplementary blocks are given, or if the drug is given intravenously. The patient may complain of perioral tingling, and become light-headed, anxious, drowsy or complain of tinnitus and may then progress to a convulsion. In the early stages, surgery should be abandoned and the patient given oxygen and small doses of benzodiazepines, e.g. midazolam in 1–2 mg increments: convulsions will require airway control, oxygen by positive pressure and anticonvulsant therapy with benzodiazepines or

in refractory cases, thiopentone. Hypotension and cardiac arrest may occur.

MINIMIZING RISKS OF LOCAL ANAESTHESIA

1 Apply basic monitoring (ECG, pulse oximetry, BP).
2 Establish IV access.
3 Have equipment and skill for cardiopulmonary resuscitation.
4 Have relevant training and knowledge for the procedure.
5 Pass the needle with the eye in the primary position.
6 Use a needle approximately 25 mm long: do not position the hub beyond the orbital rim.
7 Ensure the eye is mobile after passage of the needle.
8 Aspirate before injecting, to avoid intravascular injection.
9 Wait at least 15 minutes after performing the block, before preparation of the eye and draping the patient to ensure that there are no early complications.

SEDATION

This may be needed in very anxious patients, but for most, explanation, reassurance and a gentle touch will suffice. If sedation is used, the goal should be to provide amnesia and analgesia for any painful stages of the procedure, and to avoid having a patient sedated during surgery whose sedation may wane leading to a sudden movement occurring at a critical time. A judicious dose of midazolam IV (1–2 mg is generally enough in the elderly and its onset is slow) may be appropriate, but anaesthetists may prefer a cocktail based on midazolam, fentanyl and propofol mixtures, or similar agents.

The dangers of sedation include loss of cooperation or consciousness during surgery, partial obstruction of the airway causing snoring, total obstruction of the airway leading to hypoxia and hypercarbia, and recovery from this situation with sudden gasps and patient movement.

GENERAL ANAESTHESIA

This is now conducted with agents that are well handled by even the frail and elderly and so its use does not preclude day-case surgery, but provision for adequate recovery must be made.

Endotracheal intubation with the problems of coughing during extubation and recovery can be avoided by using the laryngeal mask airway (LMA), but this must be well positioned and secured, with adequate ventilation assured, before surgery is commenced. There is a lower incidence of postoperative sore throat after use of the LMA.

General anaesthesia should be offered when the concept of local anaesthesia is unacceptable to patient or surgeon, in those where communication is difficult due to mental disease or disability, or where there is a language barrier that prior explanation through an interpreter cannot break. An inability to lie supine for the appropriate time, as in severe cases of cardiac and respiratory disease, may need consideration of general anaesthesia, but a compromise on positioning may avoid this being necessary. Movement disorders affecting the head may necessitate the use of general anaesthesia. Allergy to local anaesthesia is reported, and this is generally to the *amide* group: it is a rare problem, but alternative ways of providing peroperative analgesia include general anaesthesia, or a topical technique as most agents used topically are of the *ester* group of local anaesthetics.

The anaesthetic induction agents (with the exception of ketamine) all lower IOP, but propofol causes a greater reduction than thiopentone. Propofol, used by continuous infusion for maintenance of anaesthesia, keeps the IOP low. A similar effect is achieved by the modern volatile anaesthetic agents, and is one of the benefits of general anaesthesia.

The choroidal blood flow is autoregulated, so, excluding extreme conditions, changes in blood pressure have no effect upon IOP, but there is a linear relationship between choroidal flow and arterial carbon dioxide tension. Hence mild hyperventilation induces choroidal vasoconstriction and lowers IOP, and can be used to good effect to soften an eye during surgery.

A well-conducted general anaesthetic not only ensures a still eye and a still patient, but will also significantly reduce IOP and may improve operating conditions. This is an important consideration when contemplating surgery on a patient in whom there had been complications at a previous operation.

COMPLICATIONS OF GENERAL ANAESTHESIA

In appropriately selected and prepared patients complications of general anaesthesia are rare, but they can occur. They include:

1 Minor trauma: damage to lips, teeth and oro-pharyngeal mucous membranes may be caused by instrumentation of the mouth during passage of endotracheal tubes or laryngeal mask airways. Simple analgesics and mouthwashes generally provide relief.

2 Stridor from laryngeal spasm: this can occur soon after extubation, and is distressing for the patient and recovery room staff. The anaesthetist should be summoned, oxygen given and the patient nursed semi-sitting: it generally settles, but some treat with nebulized adrenaline, diuretics and steroids, or other agents, and rarely the patient may need to be reintubated.

3 Respiratory muscle weakness: this is now much rarer as the modern muscle relaxants can generally be effectively reversed. While help is being obtained, the basic management is to give oxygen by facemask, and if necessary, oxygen by manual ventilation with bag and mask. This technique is part of Advanced Life Support, with which all doctors should be familiar. Do not hesitate to give oxygen, even in the patient with chronic chest disease: hypoxia kills rapidly, hypercarbia's problems develop more slowly.

POSTOPERATIVE CARE

The majority of patients can be discharged home on the day of surgery, after either LA or GA, providing adequate social support is available. If this is not available, hospital or hostel support may be required. Some mild analgesia may be needed and even modern GA may result in some nausea, requiring postoperative anti-emetics to be given. Other problems are rare.

As a local anaesthetic block wears off, approximately 4–5 hours after surgery, the patient may experience unpleasant dysaesthesia or pain. This can be alarming to the timid patient but is usually managed with reassurance and mild analgesics such as paracetamol.

Driving is to be avoided for 24 hours after a general anaesthetic, although strong evidence for this recommendation is hard to find. It should also be avoided by patients who are wearing a shield or dressing and are temporarily monocular.

RECOMMENDED READING

Johnson, R.W. and Forrest, F.C. (1994) *Local and General Anaesthesia for Ophthalmic Surgery.* Oxford: Butterworth-Heinemann Ltd.

Finucane, B.T. (1999) *Complications of Regional Anaesthesia.* Philadelphia: Churchill Livingstone.

Chapter 3

Standard surgical techniques: phacoemulsification and extracapsular cataract surgery

INTRODUCTION

Safety depends on the surgeon's ability to be able to match his or her surgical skills against the problem posed by the patient's eye. Arrogance is your greatest enemy and if you persist with a difficult eye with an inappropriate technique, the problems are less easily defended morally, ethically or medicolegally. The surgeon must be able to depend on a reproducible, reliable technique that will be adequate for the vast majority of straightforward cases.

Surgery should be performed within the competence of the surgeon and where the risk:benefit ratio favours a good outcome. This is the concept of defensive surgery. Time spent preparing yourself, the theatre staff and the patient before commencing an operation is time well spent.

There are almost as many different variations in surgical technique as there are cataract surgeons! A range of techniques will be needed to cover all surgical problems, but for most operations a sound basic technique will give reproducibly good outcomes. The techniques presented in this chapter, extracapsular surgery and phaco using 'divide and conquer', represent what the authors regard as the foundations of a good, dependable technique. It is upon these techniques that other manoeuvres can be mastered. You return to them when you in turn start teaching surgery.

The skills required to complete a phaco operation that goes wrong are based on ECCE surgery. An operation should not be started if the surgeon is not in the position to deal with the full range of potential complications. This is the enigma of the current approach to teaching cataract surgery. Trainees are taught to begin with phaco without instilling the escape skills of ECCE. For this reason, a preferred technique for ECCE is presented first.

PREOPERATIVE PREPARATION

THE SURGEON

You must be sitting comfortably to perform microsurgery. The microscope should be adjusted for your own interpupillary distance and refraction. It should be placed high enough to allow your back to be straight throughout the operation (Fig. 3.1). A hunched posture may be tolerable for a case or two but rarely for an entire list and certainly not for a lifetime of operating.

The phaco pedal will require the most precision in its control and should therefore be reserved for your dominant foot with the microscope controls at the other. The surgeon's chair should have armrests. Your forearms should be as near to horizontal as possible. This is the most ergonomically efficient position for the small muscles of the hand.

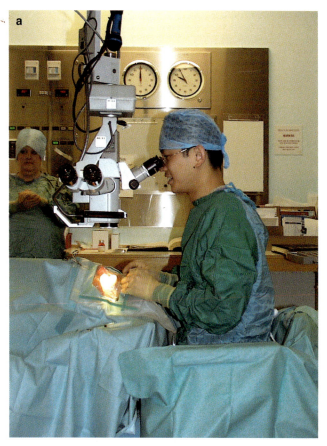
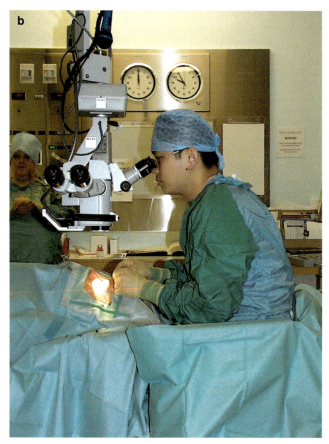

Fig 3.1 (**a**) The correct operating position; (**b**) the incorrect operating position

THE NURSE

If theatre staff are informed of potential problems in advance, appropriate additional instruments or equipment can be on hand. For example, small pupils may require stretching or the use of iris hooks, or a capsule tension ring may be needed with traumatic cataracts or where there is an unstable lens. Theatre staff always appreciate advance warning and such forward planning will facilitate the running of the list.

If there are special problems with a particular patient, go and talk directly to the theatre staff concerned. These instructions should also be included on the operating list, which will act as an *aide mémoire* for all on the day of surgery.

THE PATIENT

The patient's comfort and ease are crucial. Good relationships with the anaesthetic team will recruit their intelligent help to achieve this. Patient anxiety is reduced by having a member of staff hold the patient's hand throughout the procedure when done under local anaesthetic. The patient appreciates the human contact during the claustro-phobic time when their head is draped. A simple squeeze of the hand is sufficient to warn the attendant that the patient is uncomfortable or worried.

Elderly patients are often kyphotic and many have arthritis which can affect the neck. The use of a pillow under the patient's knees or padding around the neck may make a huge difference to their comfort (Fig. 3.2). With regard to positioning, the patient's head should be as near to the end of the table as possible and the forehead and chin should be in the same horizontal plane.

SKIN AND EYE PREPARATION

The eye is prepared by washing the skin of the lids (Fig. 3.3) and instilling 5% povidine iodine (Betadine) in aqueous solution in the fornices. The chemical takes time to penetrate the 'biofilm', and must be left in contact for approximately 5 minutes. It is our practice to ask the anaesthetist to do this after the anaesthetic has been given, before the patient is brought into the theatre.

The authors use a disposable drape that leads all fluids away from the operating field into a reservoir that hangs over the head of the operating table (Fig. 3.4). As the lids are draped, they are gently everted, capturing the lashes.

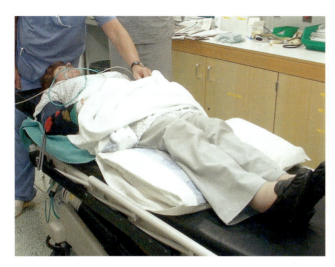

Fig. 3.2 Note the position of a pillow behind the patient's knees

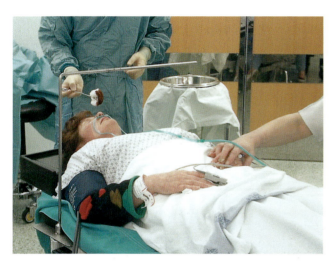

Fig. 3.3 Preparing the eye, washing the skin with povidine iodine solution

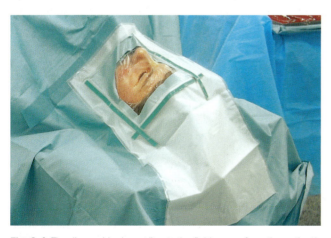

Fig. 3.4 The disposable drape directs the fluids away from the patient's head, keeping the operative field dry

The drape is incised and the lids held gently open by a speculum (Fig. 3.5). The use of a partially opaque material for the drape can reduce the claustrophobia felt by some patients.

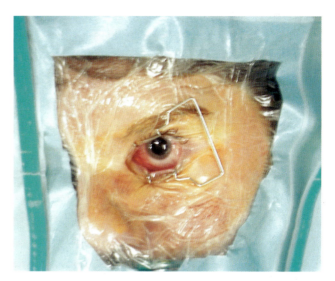

Fig. 3.5 A wire speculum is used to keep both the eye open and ensure that the drape covers the lashes and lid margins

EXTRACAPSULAR CATARACT EXTRACTION (ECCE) SURGERY

Preferred technique

The technique for extracapsular extraction of the lens employing a corneal section and the 'technique d'envelope' is presented in a step-wise fashion and illustrated with a series of diagrams.

SUPERIOR RECTUS STAY SUTURE

When using a corneal section, a superior rectus stay suture is rarely needed, but is useful when the superior rectus is active and the eye is turned up; this makes access to the superior limbus difficult. The suture can also be used in conjunction with an inferior rectus suture to bring a deep-set eye forward.

INCISION

A corneal incision is used. The length of the incision must be sufficient to allow expression of the nucleus, which will vary in size and volume, but an arc of 120° is the minimum needed.

As a general rule, dense nuclear cataracts in elderly patients have large, hard nuclei. The darker the cataract and the older the patient the larger the nucleus and the harder the lens. The younger the patient, the smaller the nucleus and adolescents and children will probably have no nucleus at all (and require tiny incisions for their removal and can thus just be aspirated). For most cataracts, the internal opening will need to be of the order of 10 mm. Remember that it is better to have a larger wound through which to deliver the lens than an incision which is too small and which obstructs the passage of nucleus.

The curvature of the wound can be marked on the cornea with the tip of a diamond knife. Try to keep this arc as concentric as possible (Fig. 3.6).

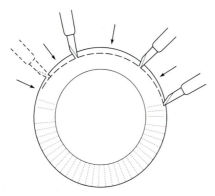

Fig. 3.6 Planned corneal incision: note that the length of the incision is approximately 120°

A 'grab' point is made at one end of the section by a partial thickness stab with the diamond knife. The eye can be held here when cutting the section (Fig. 3.7).

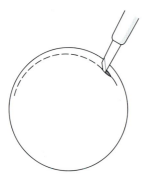

Fig. 3.7 Making a 'grab' point with a diamond knife, partially penetrating the cornea at the start of the incision

Aim to make the incision double bevelled in cross-section, with the first cut aimed backwards to the centre of the eye, and the second at right-angles to this, aiming towards the centre of the pupil. A partial thickness groove is cut running just inside the limbal arcade with the blade angled at the centre of the eye (this will almost feel like cutting 'backwards') (Fig. 3.8).

The angle of the blade is altered so that the plane of its cut is now aimed at the centre of the pupillary plane. The

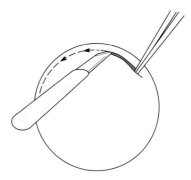

Fig. 3.8 Holding the cornea with forceps and cutting the first, partial thickness groove. Note the angle of the blade

section is deepened until aqueous is seen to leak and then completed by running the tip of the diamond in a continuous smooth movement from the centre of the wound to each end of the incision (Fig. 3.9).

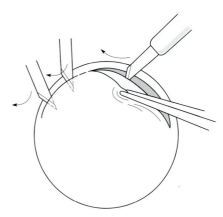

Fig. 3.9 Completing the section by changing the angle of the cut to make a bevelled incision

Fill the anterior chamber with viscoelastic. Pass the Rycroft cannula across the eye to the opposite corneoscleral angle before injecting. As the viscoelastic is introduced aqueous will be forced out through the section (Fig. 3.10). The cornea will not now collapse as you carry out the next intraocular manoeuvres.

CAPSULOTOMY

Start the capsulotomy by making a small, horizontal cut in the capsule with the cystotome, approximately one-third of the way down the lens (Fig. 3.11). This is then extended medially and laterally under the iris (Fig. 3.12). The nucleus can be freed by hydrodissection but this is not usually necessary.

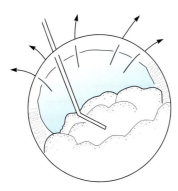

Fig. 3.10 Filling the anterior chamber with viscoelastic

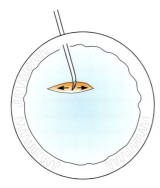

Fig. 3.11 Starting an 'envelope' capsulotomy one-third of the way down the anterior capsule

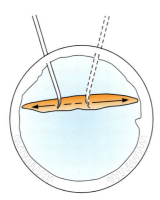

Fig. 3.12 Extending the capsulotomy laterally and medially under the iris

NUCLEUS EXPRESSION

Nucleus expression is accomplished in three quite separate movements which together tilt, prolapse, push and deliver the nucleus. With a pair of toothed or grooved forceps grasp the posterior lip of the superior limbus approximately 4 mm behind the limbus, and press towards the centre of the eye (Fig. 3.13). This will tilt the upper pole of the lens forwards and the upper capsular leaf will be seen to retract over the equator of the lens. As it starts to

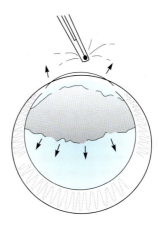

Fig. 3.13 Nucleus expression – step 1

move through the capsular opening and pupil, the section will gape.

With forceps, now push on the eye inferiorly, applying counter pressure which will ensure continued progress of the nucleus (Fig. 3.14). The forces from the two hands should be steady and balanced but varied as necessary to steer and nudge the lens through the corneal wound and out of the eye. By an alternately rocking pressure between the upper and lower forceps, even a large lens can be encouraged out of the eye (Fig. 3.15).

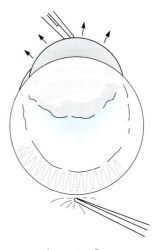

Fig. 3.14 Nucleus expression – step 2

The prolapsed nucleus is gently brushed aside with either forceps or a sponge and the anterior chamber immediately reformed with balanced salt solution (BSS) (Fig. 3.16).

CORTICAL TOILET

Aspirate the soft lens matter (SLM) using a Simcoe cannula (rather than using the I/A from a phaco machine, which is

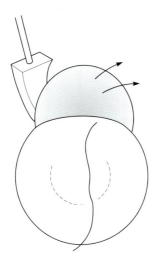

Fig. 3.15 Nucleus expression – step 3

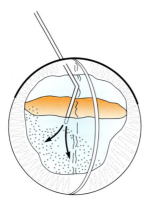

Fig. 3.16 Reforming the anterior chamber with BSS

not as easy to control in an open eye). It is easier to see where the I/A cannula is in relation to the capsule if the opening to the sac is cleared first (Fig. 3.17).

Using the pupil margin as a guide, the I/A cannula is now moved around inside the capsule, methodically grasp-

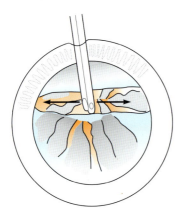

Fig. 3.17 Clearing the opening of the capsular bag

ing, then aspirating the epinucleus and soft lens matter (the cornea and iris are protected from the I/A by the anterior capsule) (Fig. 3.18). If the capsule catches in the aspiration port, release the suction and it should fall away; or squeeze the plunger of the syringe to regurgitate the capsule.

To remove the SLM from the upper fornix of the bag, the Simcoe is turned onto its side so that the aspirating port directly engages the SLM (Fig. 3.19); some surgeons advocate aspirating this more difficult area first.

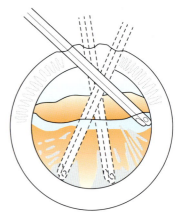

Fig. 3.18 Aspirating soft lens matter

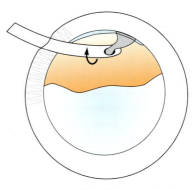

Fig. 3.19 Clearing the upper third of the capsular bag. Note that the Simcoe cannula is rotated so that the aspiration port engages the SLM

When the capsule is clear of all cortical material, viscoelastic is injected into the bag to splint it open and receive the IOL (Fig. 3.20).

LENS IMPLANTATION

A single-piece, all PMMA lens, 13.5 mm in length should be used. The lens is grasped at its proximal edge with the MacPhearson's forceps aligned along its longitudinal axis. The leading haptic is delivered into the capsular envelope, and well into the capsule (Fig. 3.21). Once the maximum diameter of the IOL has entered the eye ('crowning'), the lens is released and the forceps removed from the eye.

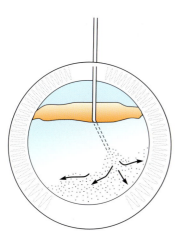

Fig. 3.20 Injecting viscoelastic into the empty capsular bag

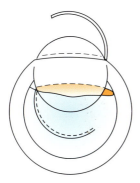

Fig. 3.21 Inserting the leading haptic into the capsular bag, the lens is held with MacPhearson's forceps

The trailing haptic is placed into the upper sac by taking the tip of the haptic and pushing it into the eye whilst pronating the hand. This is an awkward manoeuvre for left-handed surgeons who can use a Kuglan hook to simply position the upper loop instead (Fig. 3.22).

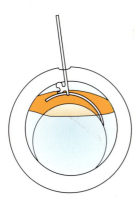

Fig. 3.22 Completing implantation. The upper haptic is placed in the upper fornix of the sac using a Kuglan hook

COMPLETION OF ANTERIOR CAPSULECTOMY

The anterior capsule must be removed from the visual axis because it is cellular and will opacify. Having refilled the anterior chamber, two linear cuts are made in the anterior capsule using long, fine scissors (Fig. 3.23).

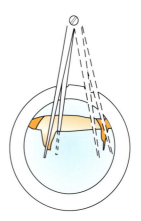

Fig. 3.23 Cutting two snicks in the anterior capsule

Using MacPhearson's or Utratta's forceps, take one of the free corners of capsule and tear it down and around to join up with the other incision. If the capsule seems reluctant to tear, or if the tear seems to want to follow a different direction, let the capsule go and, having injected more viscoelastic, take the other tag and tear in the opposite direction to meet the original tear. The eye is now ready to be sutured and the operation completed (Fig. 3.24).

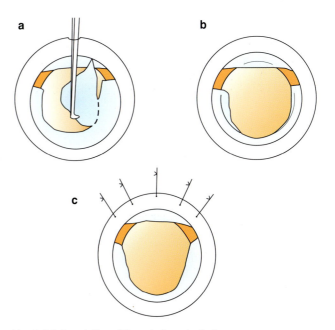

Fig. 3.24 Completion of the anterior capsulectomy

SUTURING

The corneal wound is now closed with 10/0 nylon using either continuous or interrupted sutures. If interrupted sutures are used, at least 5 sutures will be required; if a continuous suture is used at least 7 bites will be needed to close the wound. Reform the anterior chamber with BSS. If the wound is watertight it will not leak. If the wound is not watertight, either insert further interrupted stitches or tighten the continuous suture.

If you are practised, continuous sutures are quicker to place than interrupted. The tension forces of the suture are spread equally along the section. Induced astigmatism is easily seen and can be adjusted by tightening or loosening the suture before tying the final knot. On the other hand, if this suture needs to be removed, e.g. to relieve astigmatism postoperatively, the whole suture has to come out and some argue that this is a disadvantage.

Technique for continuous suture The knots of the continuous suture must be buried at either end of the wound. The suture will make a neat saw-tooth pattern along the wound. Use a 10/0 nylon suture on a cutting, spatulated needle, starting at one end of the section.

The first pass of the needle is from the floor of the section, through the scleral cornea (Fig. 3.25a). The needle is then passed through from the corneal side back into the floor of the section and tied with a surgical knot (3:1:1 throws) (Fig. 3.25b, c). The knot will be seen to lie in the wound and not be lying proud on the surface.

Continue the suturing, starting the next pass of the needle from the deep surface of the wound (Fig. 3.25d). Having brought the needle out on the sceral side of the wound, the suture progresses along the length of the wound in a series of bites which pass through both corneal and scleral edges of the wound. This is continued to the end of the section (Fig. 3.25e). Each pass of the needle should be at an equal angle to a radian passing from the centre of the cornea through the apex of the stitch creating a neat saw-tooth pattern (Fig. 3.25f). The forces induced by the sutures are thus equally distributed and any tendency of the cornea to shear against the sclera is restricted.

To tie the buried knot at the distal end of the wound, the needle is passed back on itself, i.e. from the proximal side to exit in the floor of the section, and the suture is then tied on itself by bringing up a loop of suture from the floor of the wound (Fig. 3.25g, h). A double throw is placed on the suture (Fig. 3.25i), but before completing the knot inflate the A/C with BSS (Fig. 3.25j), aspirate all remaining viscoelastic with the Simcoe cannula and tighten the continuous thread. Start from the distal end of the suture and work towards the untied end (Fig. 3.25k).

Once the suture has been tightened there should be neither leak nor slack. Any folding of the cornea related to the sutures should be noted. If this is marked, the suture is too tight and should be eased slightly from the incomplete knot. Once you are happy with the tension of the

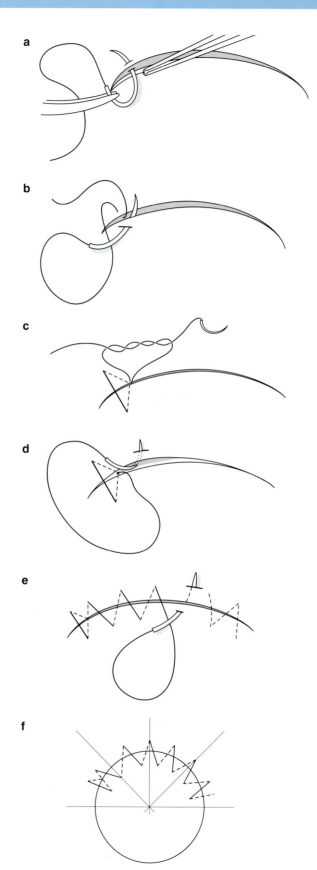

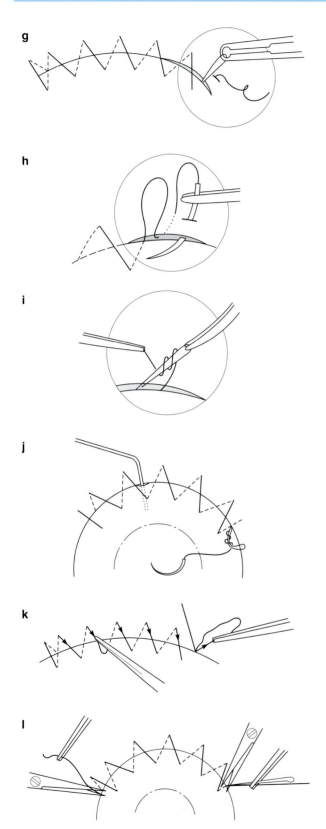

g

h

i

j

k

l

Fig. 3.25 Technique for continuous suturing of a cataract section with 10/0 nylon. Note the knots are buried at both ends and the sutures form a neat saw-tooth pattern

suture, two further individual throws can be laid which will complete the knot. The suture ends should be trimmed and buried within the section (Fig. 3.25l).

Interrupted sutures   This is an alternative method for closing the eye. The sutures take longer to do than a continuous and must be tied individually which makes it harder to get an even tension in the wound; this increases the risk of astigmatism. The use of a 'tatting' knot is a good way of controlling tightness; each suture can be locked like this until the whole wound is sewn up and then the knots are completed when the tension is even (Fig. 3.26). The advantage of using interrupted sutures lies in being able to adjust wound tightness postoperatively by selective suture removal.

If the time taken to suture is likely to be prolonged (e.g. because of inexperience), protect the macula from the axial illumination of the microscope by using either a square of sponge material or a blob of viscoelastic on the cornea.

Re-inflate the eye and then aspirate the remaining viscoelastic with the Simcoe cannula, passed between two sutures. Retest for water-tightness by injecting BSS through a fine Rycroft cannula and wiping the section gently with a sponge. Rotate the knots of the sutures so that they lie buried within the substance of the wound and do not cause irritation (Fig. 3.27). Replace any sutures that seem loose after this or place further stitches if the wound continues to leak.

A subconjunctival injection of antibiotic is given; cefuroxime (125 mg) has a broad spectrum of activity, and does not have such toxic affects on the conjunctiva as subconjunctival gentamicin.

HEALING OF ECCE WOUNDS

The principles of wound edge apposition are crucial whether closing the eye with interrupted or continuous sutures. Whichever technique is chosen, a corneal incision must be supported by sutures for at least 12 weeks or significant postoperative ATR astigmatism will quickly develop. Shorter wounds, e.g. those used for secondary lens implants, need less time (approx. 8 weeks) for stability. The temptation to remove corneal sutures to treat astigmatism should be resisted until this critical period of healing is over. This delay may seem inordinate when one's experience is solely that of phacoemulsification with its instantaneous visual rehabilitation.

PHACOEMULSIFICATION

Introduction

The transmitted energy of ultrasound causes cavitation and fragmentation of the crystalline lens. With this primary observation and development of the technology by

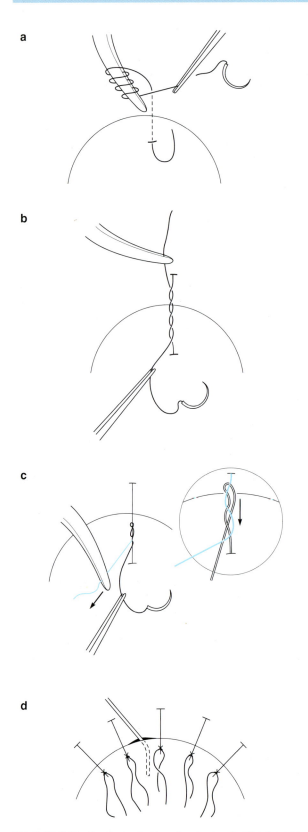

Fig. 3.26 Tatting knot, showing how the short end of the thread is brought down on the knot whilst the long end is held under tension. The knot will hold itself

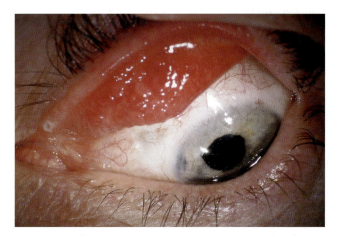

Fig. 3.27 Papillary conjunctivitis caused by protruding suture ends

Charles Kelman, small incision cataract surgery has pushed forward dramatically. Phacoemulsification is now the most commonly performed method of removing cataracts in the developed world.

The techniques of the surgery are varied and the chosen technique may apparently vary considerably from one surgeon to the next. Certainly the techniques have become much more refined and therefore also easier to perform and teach. For the newcomer to phaco-cataract surgery this spread of technique will seem daunting and may make it difficult to know which route or method to choose.

The principles, however, are the same. Energy is delivered to the lens by way of a probe which is tuned to oscillate at ultrasonic frequencies. By directing this energy within the eye, the surgeon is able to carve up the cataractous lens. The liquefied residuum is removed by the rapid exchange of irrigation fluid with the lens 'milk'. The small incision allows rapid visual rehabilitation postoperatively.

Phaco equipment

It is crucial that the machine you use is reliable and that you are entirely *au fait* with its performance characteristics. The characteristics of each phaco are different. Some are simple, others much more complex but all allow you to adjust the rate of fluid exchange, the power of the probe and the level of vacuum required for surgery. Most have in-built controls that prevent sudden collapse of the anterior chamber during lens removal and are much easier and safer to use than early models. It is important that surgeons fully understand the settings and characteristics of the particular machine they will use in their operating theatre. It must be realized that it will take time to tune the machine to each surgeon's preferred approach to phaco. It is therefore beyond the scope of this book to do anything other than state the principles of the surgery rather than categorically state exact settings for the many sorts of phaco machine in use.

PROGRAMME SETTINGS AND EXTERNAL CONTROLS

The levels of vacuum, aspiration flow rate and phacoemulsification are usually set in a series of programmes (one, two and three). Each will have a group of pre-set levels and each of these programmes are used in order to complete the different stages of the operation.

The pedal has three basic positions which activate the probe functions: 1 – infusion; 2 – aspiration; 3 – phaco power. As the pedal is depressed to position 1, the pinch valve opens, allowing the infusion fluid to flow into the eye. In position 2, the aspiration starts and the influx and removal of BSS should be in balance. In position 3, the needle begins to oscillate, producing 'phaco power'. In parallel with this, vacuum and phaco power are available progressively as the pedal is further depressed.

A further position, not to be forgotten, is 'reflux', which can be invaluable in regurgitating tissues and capsule if they have been unintentionally caught in the probe. The position of this pedal or direction of movement varies from machine to machine.

FLUIDICS

The safety of phaco surgery requires that the variables of flow, vacuum, intraocular pressure and phaco power be delivered in an appropriate and expected way. The irrigating fluid will remove the lens debris, the vacuum will let you hold portions of the lens, and the power or energy of the phaco tip will carve and dissolve the lens. The equipment allows these to be varied to your needs, but when first starting phaco, it is difficult to understand the implications of so many settings and to understand what levels are needed and why. Each variable can be considered individually.

Intraocular pressure   Intraocular tension is controlled by bottle height. This may be varied and is independent of the machinery. If the bottle is too high, there will be a tendency for the iris to prolapse; if too low, the anterior chamber will tend to collapse as vacuum is applied.

Vacuum   Vacuum is generated either by a peristaltic or a venturi pump, and each make of machine will have one or the other. The different ways of producing the vacuum give the machines quite different performance profiles.

Peristaltic pumps produce vacuum only when the tip of the phaco or I/A cannula is occluded. Then, and only then, will the vacuum rise to its pre-set maximum. The time taken for the vacuum to rise from zero to its pre-set maximum is called the vacuum rise time (VRT). Some machines also have an automated VRT. This can be set to cut in once the vacuum reaches a pre-determined threshold. A slow VRT prevents high vacuums from building quickly, which is useful when learning phaco. There is

also less risk of anterior chamber collapse once occlusion is broken.

The VRT can be reduced if the surgeon is attempting a delicate manoeuvre such as posterior capsular polishing.

Venturi pumps on the other hand produce vacuum constantly, whether the tip of the probe is occluded or not. There is therefore no pressure rise time, the vacuum is instantly present. Things happen quickly and lens material or vital tissue such as iris or capsule is readily incarcerated. This characteristic is useful in the technique of 'phaco-chop' where the lens fragments are held by the vacuum as the chopper is used to cleave the nucleus.

They seem easy to use because the vacuum is so good at grabbing and holding things, but it is not always possible to see or control what else has been grabbed or held!

Flow rate   Aspiration flow rate (AFR) is changeable only on the peristaltic machines. It has a pre-set maximum for each programme. Increasing the AFR induces a current in the eye which will carry lens matter towards the port, producing similar characteristics to a venturi machine; a higher AFR setting in programme 3 is used to move cortical or soft lens matter to the phaco needle. In the venturi machines, the vacuum is always 'sucking' the fluid out of the eye inducing its own current, tugging at any loose or moveable tissue.

Phaco power   The potential power in the tip of a phaco machine is considerable, but the power needed to remove the lens is, however, much less than the maximum available. Phaco power is increased steadily as the foot switch is depressed in position 3 (linear phaco). Use the least power possible to carve the lens. The phaco tip should pass through the lens with minimal rocking of the nucleus. If the nucleus rolls away from the tip without cutting, that movement will place a strain on the suspensory ligaments of the lens.

Remember that the probe passes through the lens in the pathway cut by cavitation in front of the vibrating tip and not like a knife. Pushing harder on the nucleus will not make it cut faster or better; rather it will strain the zonule or tear the capsule. Enough power must be generated at the tip of the needle to make the nucleus disintegrate. If the probe fails to cut the nucleus in spite of fully depressing the pedal, a higher maximum will have to be used, e.g. if the maximum pre-set power is 50%, increase this to 60% or 70% and see if this cuts the lens.

In eyes with very dense, hard lenses, a high setting will be needed to get through the nucleus, as will be the case where zonular weakness is suspected, e.g. pseudoexfoliation syndrome. Lower power settings are used for cataracts in young adults or when removing the epinucleus.

Less power is needed to scoop the soft superficial cortex, but as the probe moves to the centre of the lens, greater energy is needed where the nuclear density is greatest. Similarly, as the carving progresses to the deepest layers, the power required to carve will be less and less.

Once the lens has been broken into smaller pieces (by fractis or by the nuclear chopper), the pieces are removed by the phaco probe, which works best on harder fragments when the energy is delivered in a series of pulses or bursts of phaco power. The fragments are held on the tip as the pieces of lens are dragged into the mouth of the instrument.

All parameters can and should be altered to suit the case and the technique being used. As experience grows, the surgeon will become more comfortable at making these adjustments and understanding how and why they should be varied.

SURGICAL TECHNIQUES OF PHACOEMULSIFICATION

There are many ways of performing phacoemulsification. Some of the names given to the techniques are colourful, others are confusing. One reliable method, recommended for learning phaco, is 'divide and conquer' or 'nuclear fractis'. The operation is broken down into a series of deliberate, key steps which underline the strategic principles of small incision cataract surgery. Each of the steps must be mastered. The technique is easy to teach and learn and, except for the most difficult cases, is a reliable method for removing cataracts. Other techniques, such as nuclear chopping, can be learned later and adapted as skills and confidence grow.

STAY SUTURES

The bi-manual manipulations of phaco allow control of the position and movements of the eye. A superior rectus stay suture is therefore rarely required, but can be useful in eyes that are turned upwards as a result of either an unbalanced local anaesthetic block or when a light general anaesthetic is used.

Similarly, where the eye is deep set in the orbit, the use of combined inferior and superior rectus sutures (6/0 prolene on a round-bodied needle) will lift the eye anteriorly, improving access and drainage of fluids.

PREOPERATIVE CHECKS

Before starting to operate, the surgeon should check that the machine is working satisfactorily and that the settings are appropriate for the case (Box 3.1).

INCISION

Whereas ECCE is an 'open' operation, phacoemulsification is a 'closed' eye operation. There is neither direct visualization of the anterior segment structures nor is the eye opened to deliver the lens. Operative visualization is

---

Box 3.1 Checking the phaco machine

▶ Is the probe correctly joined to the irrigating and aspirating tubing?

▶ Does the irrigation fluid emerge when the peddle is depressed?

▶ Does the probe tune properly?

▶ Does the BSS readily reflux? This lifeline is a good final check that all is well with the machinery and that the technical checks are satisfactory

---

through the cornea and all manipulations take place under its dome, the shape of which must be maintained.

During phaco, instruments are restricted to arcs of movement by the incisions which act as fulcrums for these movements. Clumsy manipulations will distort the cornea and reduce visibility.

Principles of phaco wounds Incisions have two dimensions, circumferential width and radial length. Size matters; the phaco incision should be wide enough to allow instruments in and out of the eye, and also to permit fluid to pass down the outside of the infusion sleeve, thus cooling the probe and maintaining the temperature of the ocular tissues at safe levels.

If the wound is *too wide*, or poorly constructed, fluid will pour out around the phaco probe. This disrupts the balance of aspiration and infusion, leading to marked fluctuation in anterior chamber depth. Delicate manipulations of lens, capsule and cortex then become difficult to control.

If the wound is *too narrow*, it will be difficult to move the instruments in and out of the eye, the cornea will distort in an unacceptable way reducing visibility, or the wound will be heated by the phaco-probe causing a burn. Similar problems occur if the length of the tunnel is *too long*. The use of a diamond or disposable keratome of the correct size for the instruments that need to pass through the wound ensures good construction.

The incisions should be directed so that they aim towards the centre of the lens and let the instruments lie comfortably in the hand when the tips are in the eye (Fig. 3.28a, b). In this way you can minimize wound distortion and maximize efficient working in the anterior chamber.

The largest object that will pass through the incision is the IOL, and the wound must be large enough, or enlarged to accept that lens. If a large lens is to be inserted, e.g. a one-piece all PMMA lens, then a phaco tunnel is a better wound to use because it can be enlarged without loss of stability and if less than 6 mm will not have to be sutured.

Whenever an instrument is removed from the eye and at the end of the operation, the wound should be sufficiently well constructed to self-seal. This stability contributes greatly to minimizing postoperative astigmatism. If the

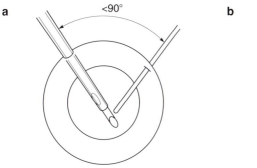
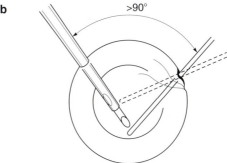

Fig. 3.28 Correct (**a**) and incorrect (**b**) axis for second incision

wound has had to be enlarged to accept the IOL it may be too long and not watertight. Compared to the corneal 'stab', the enlargement is less well controlled.

At the end of the operation the wound must be watertight, and if there is any doubt as to the integrity of the wound, it should be sutured.

Recommended incision techniques

Phaco incisions are either 'clear corneal' or through a 'phaco tunnel'. Either technique is acceptable provided the principles stated above are respected.

Clear corneal incisions are quicker and easier to perform and do not require diathermy. They may induce more astigmatism and occasionally need suturing. They are more easily made at the top of the eye when learning surgery. Later, as skills improve, the temporal approach can be adopted if preferred.

Phaco tunnels may take a little longer to create and require diathermy to control bleeding, but they induce less astigmatism and rarely need suturing even when enlarged to 5.5 mm to accept a one-piece PMMA IOL. The tissue posterior to the limbus heals quicker because they are vascular and finally, it is easier to convert to an ECCE section if problems are encountered when teaching.

CONSTRUCTING A CLEAR CORNEAL WOUND

A 4.00 mm length is marked with callipers at the superior limbus between 1 and 2 o'clock or 10 and 11 o'clock if the surgeon is left-handed. If a stepped incision is wanted, a shallow, partial thickness incision is now cut with a diamond knife, into clear cornea. You should aim for no more than one-third thickness.

A keratome of the recommended size, e.g. 3.2 mm, is now passed into the eye in a plane parallel to the iris (Fig. 3.29a). This will create a shelving, self-sealing wound (Fig. 3.29b, c). As the tip of the blade enters the eye, you will note the internal opening in Descemet's membrane. The paracentesis for the second instrument is created using a stab incision with a diamond blade (Fig. 3.29d).

CONSTRUCTING A PHACO TUNNEL WOUND

These wounds are best made superiorly, at either 10.30 o'clock or 1.30 o'clock for left-handers. A superior rectus suture (6/0 prolene on a needle point 1/2 circle needle) may help to stop the eye rotating when dissecting the tunnel and improve exposure.

The limbal conjunctiva is reflected with fine spring scissors, over an arc of about 6 mm (Fig. 3.30a). A cord length

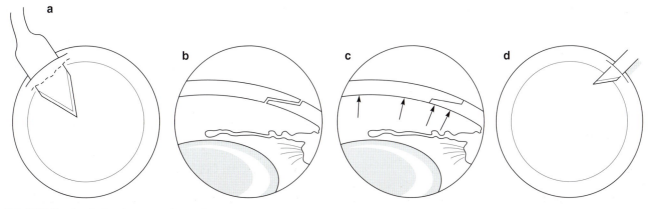

Fig. 3.29 Constructing a clear corneal wound

of 5.5 mm is measured, 2.0 mm posterior to the limbus. Any bleeding vessels *behind* this line should be gently cauterized. Do not cauterize in front of this line or the strength of the roof of the phaco tunnel will be weakened.

A diamond or crescent blade is used to make a partial thickness incision in the shape of a reverse smile (Fig. 3.30b). You should aim for a depth similar to the superficial incision used for a trabeculectomy.

The crescent blade is now used to burrow forwards, towards and under the limbus, keeping the depth sufficiently shallow to be able to visualize the knife under the tunnel roof (Fig. 3.30c). The angle of dissection is parallel to the sclera. The whole tunnel should be undermined equally as it extends into the peripheral cornea.

When the dissection has extended far enough onto the cornea (i.e. the crescent blade is just visible under the vascular arcade of the peripheral cornea), a keratome is used to enter the eye. As the tip of the blade engages the distal

end of the tunnel, its heel should be lifted and the cornea will be seen to dimple (Fig. 3.30d). If this sign is not seen the tunnel should be extended further forward with the crescent blade. Aim the tip towards the centre of the CCC (continuous curvilinear capsulorrhexis, see below) as the keratome opens the wound.

Once the incision has been made, the eye is filled with viscoelastic (Fig. 3.30e). The viscoelastic cannula is advanced across the eye to the 6 o'clock position injecting viscoelastic as it proceeds and displacing the aqueous that will escape around the cannula as it lies in the wound.

Continuous curvilinear capsulorrhexis (CCC)

CCC is a crucial stage of the operation. The size of the tear should be small enough to prevent forward displacement of the lens and yet big enough to allow cortical aspiration and insertion of the IOL. The CCC should be central and overlap the edge of the optic of the IOL at the end of the operation.

In young patients, the elasticity of the zonule and capsule together produce a tendency for uncontrolled tear as you try to do the CCC. In these eyes ample viscoelastic must be used to push the lens backwards and relieve the distracting forces of the zonule, which threaten to induce a dramatic extension of the CCC tear. Re-fill the AC with viscoelastic whenever the tear threatens to extend outwards under the iris.

MAKING A CYSTOTOME FOR CAPSULORRHEXIS

The ready-made proprietary cystotomes have a long tip which digs deeply into the underlying cortical material as the initial capsulotomy is made. This can make it difficult to see the capsular edge and spoil the start of the CCC. However, using a 27G hypodermic needle, a cystotome with a much smaller and precise tip can be easily fashioned. The tip will be large enough to pierce the capsule but not so long as to disturb the underlying cortical fibres.

The needle is mounted on a 2 ml syringe. Turn the tip bevel down on to a flat metallic surface such as a Bard–Parker handle (Fig. 3.31a), and lift the syringe bending the tip through about 75°. The tip of the needle will be seen to form a small hook (Fig. 3.31b).

With Castroviejo's needle holders, gently bend the shaft of the needle in a counter curve (Fig. 3.31c).

The needle holders are repositioned half way down the needle's shaft and twisted sharply to produce a 120° angle on the bevelled side (Fig. 3.31d).

TEARING THE CCC

The technique of tearing the CCC is described below and illustrated by a series of staged drawings.

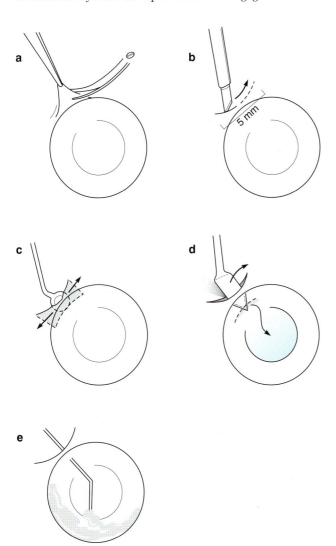

Fig. 3.30 Constructing a phaco tunnel with crescent blade and keratome

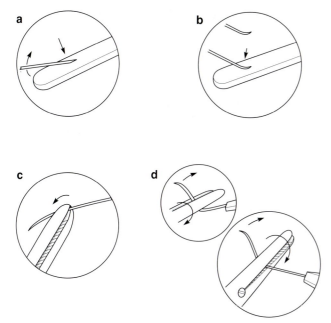

Fig. 3.31 Making a small-hook cystotome from a 27G needle

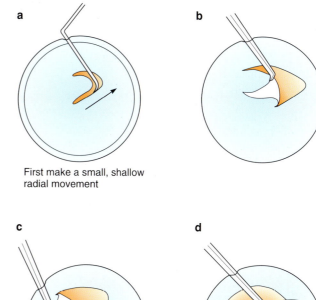

First make a small, shallow radial movement

Fig. 3.32 Tearing a CCC

With the eye filled with viscoelastic, the cystotome is inserted into the anterior chamber. Start the capsulotomy just proximal to the centre of the pupil and to the side of the microscope light reflex. The very tip of the cystotome cuts into the capsule and this tear is then drawn radially for a short distance (Fig. 3.32a).

The tear is now dragged so that it begins to run in a circumferential route (counter-clockwise or clockwise depending on whether the surgeon is left- or right-handed) until the tear is C-shaped (Fig. 3.32b). Take care not to dig the tip too deeply into the superficial lens cortex or the reflections will confuse the edge of the capsulorrhexis for the lens fibres as you attempt to extend the CCC.

Take hold of this flap of capsule with Utratta's forceps and extend the tear around the edge of the pupil (Fig. 3.32c). The folded edge can be used as a guide to the radius of the circle to be torn. Change the hold on the leading edge at regular intervals and stay close to the apex of the tear in order to control the direction of the CCC (Fig. 3.32d).

Control the capsular tear in the same way as a dog on a walk is kept in check by using a short leash; if the distance between the forceps and the point of tearing becomes too long, the tear may begin to drift dangerously to disappear behind the iris.

As the leading edge returns on itself toward the start point of the CCC, the forceps should pull towards the centre of the pupil. This ensures the tear joins up with the start point and completes the capsulorrhexis. The CCC should end in either a smooth curve or with heart-shaped dimple pointing to the centre of the CCC. If the join ends up as a V with its apex pointing outwards, there is a risk that it will extend into a radial tear.

The CCC should be approximately 4–5 mm in diameter, depending on the IOL to be inserted.

If loss of control of the tearing of the CCC threatens, re-fill the anterior chamber with viscoelastic and try again. Remember to change the position of the forceps so that they are as close to the point of tearing as possible. If sight of the flap of the tear is lost, inject further viscoelastic to help visualize it.

Second incision/paracentesis

A second incision is made to take the manipulating instruments that will be used to rotate, chop, hold or remove the nucleus. The incision also acts as a port for the viscoelastic and BSS. Positioning it is important because it will take the instruments that are held in the non-dominant hand; it should be angled to help with the several bimanual manoeuvres that will be undertaken.

This incision is made at an early stage of the operation, using a diamond blade (preferably) or the tip of the keratome. It is created with a diamond blade, positioned 75° around from the phaco wound (clockwise for a right-hander), aiming at the centre of the lens.

Hydrodelineation and hydrodissection

All phaco techniques require the lens material to be separated from the capsule so that the lens can be manipulated and removed (Fig. 3.33). The process of separation with BSS is known as hydrodissection. A useful further step, hydrodelineation, cleaves the lens nucleus from its epinucleus leaving a smaller nucleus for removal. Less energy is required to remove this smaller nucleus (Table 3.1). The epinuclear shell acts as a buffer protecting the posterior capsule (which is useful for teaching purposes). The remaining cortical shell is easily removed after the nucleus.

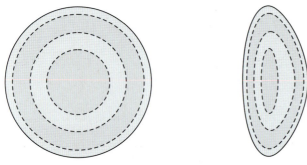

Fig. 3.33 A cross-section of the lens shows its many layers but particularly the nucleus, epinucleus and cortex. Preoperative evaluation should indicate the size and hardness of the nucleus to be expected. Hydrodelineation will confirm this impression. Be prepared to modify the surgical approach according to the findings

HYDRODELINEATION TECHNIQUE

A flat-tipped and spatulated cannula is mounted on to a 2 ml syringe filled with BSS. The tip of the cannula is pushed directly into the substance of the cortex as it crosses over the edge of the capsulorrhexis (Fig. 3.34a).

Injecting BSS in a series of tiny squirts, the cannula is advanced into the nucleus. The denser layers of the lens will separate from the jelly-like cortex. A golden coloured

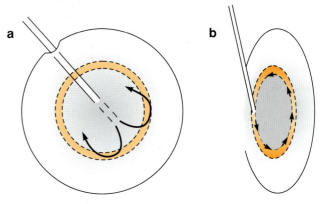

Fig. 3.34 Hydrodelineation

ring will usually be seen as the nucleus is defined. This is hydrodelineation (Fig. 3.34b).

HYDRODISSECTION TECHNIQUE

The cannula is partially withdrawn and re-directed under the farther edge of the CCC. The edge of the CCC is lifted slightly and BSS injected as the tip advances (Fig. 3.35a). A

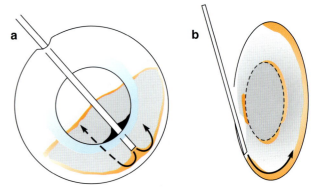

Fig. 3.35 Hydrodissection of the lens from the cortex and capsule

Table 3.1 Learning to anticipate grades of difficulty for different nucleus types			
Nucleus type		**Technique**	**Grade of difficulty**
Small nucleus	Hard	Phaco divide and conquer	Easy
	Soft	Phaco divide and conquer	Easy
Medium nucleus	Hard	Phaco divide and conquer/phaco-chop	Easy
	Soft	Phaco divide and conquer	Easy
Large nucleus	Hard (usually)	Phaco divide and conquer	Prolonged, difficult
		Phaco-chop	Quicker, moderate
	Hard	Phaco-chop	Difficult
	Very hard	Phaco-chop	Very difficult

wave of BSS should be seen to pass behind the nucleus if the lens is not too opaque (Fig. 3.35b). The lens wave will be seen to move forwards in the capsule as the fluid runs behind the lens and its capsule. If the lens comes forward, it should be balloted gently back into place. A cannula shaped like an 'umbrella handle' can be used to hydrodissect the 12 o'clock position (this is particularly useful with soft lenses that may be difficult to rotate).

The hydrodissection cannula can be used to check for free rotation of the nucleus before commencing phacoemulsification. If the nucleus will not rotate, repeat the steps of hydrodissection.

Phacoemulsification by 'divide and conquer'

Two of the principal methods of phacoemulsification, 'divide and conquer' (nuclear fractis) and 'phaco-chop', require the lens to be mechanically broken into small pieces so that the phaco can homogenize and remove the lens matter. Large, hard lenses need longer and hence more energy to remove the bits; a phaco-chopper is an efficient and safe way of quickly breaking up such nuclei, producing chunks without the need for extended bursts of energy.

The four definitive steps of this operation are nuclear sculpting, fragment removal, epinuclear removal and cortical toilet. The first three are done with the phaco probe and the last with the I/A cannula. Each of these steps has a particular group of settings on the machine; these groups are called 'programmes'.

NUCLEAR FRACTIS

The phaco is set on programme 1 – high power, low flow and low vacuum. The soft cortex and epinucleus within the CCC are removed first (Fig. 3.36a), carving a bowl in the anterior cortex.

Two grooves, which cross at right-angles to each other, are made with the phaco probe. The groove is deepened and then the nucleus is dialled around with the manipulating instrument. As each groove is deepened, the nucleus is again rotated and the process is repeated. Eventually (Fig. 3.36b) a central red reflex is seen (if the lens is hard, screw in the sleeve to allow more tip to protrude in order to reach the bottom of the trough). Make each groove as tight and as neat as possible; wide grooves are more difficult to fracture. Once a central red reflex is seen it is now time to break the nucleus into bits.

Place the phaco tip and the manipulator into the base of the groove, and then, gently moving the tips apart (Fig. 3.36c), crack the nucleus. If this action is unsuccessful, it is worth deepening the groove further and then retrying.

The action is repeated four times: the lens is rotated by 90° with the second instrument and the next groove is cracked. The splits should join up at the centre of the

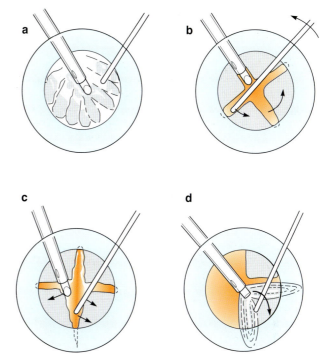

Fig. 3.36 (**a**) Central bowl in the anterior cortex; (**b**) rotating the nucleus and cutting the second groove; (**c**) cracking the nucleus; (**d**) impaling a nuclear fragment and drawing it centrally

cross that has been created and each quadrant should be independent of the other pieces.

REMOVAL OF THE NUCLEAR FRAGMENTS

The nuclear quadrants are then individually emulsified and aspirated. This phase requires higher vacuum and phaco power in 'pulse' mode to ensure efficient removal of the pieces. The machine is set to programme 2 – high vacuum, high flow, high power.

The first quadrant is tilted backwards with the manipulator so that its deepest part presents forwards (Fig. 3.36d). The phaco probe is now buried into this using a short burst of phaco power and held in place by the vacuum. Most machines emit an audible tone when the phaco tip is occluded and the vacuum is building up. The quadrant can be pulled centrally where it can be safely emulsified.

Emulsification of fragments should be done centrally where the anterior chamber is deepest and where there is less chance of aspirating capsule and iris. The second instrument can be used to squash and break up the fragment as it is held on the probe.

Repeat this for the remaining three quadrants. As the last fragment is tackled, the posterior capsule will tend to come forwards. Prevent this from being caught in the phaco probe by interposing the second instrument between the capsule and the probe as the last vestige of nucleus disappears up the phaco.

REMOVAL OF EPINUCLEUS

At the end of nuclear removal a shell of epinucleus and cortex will remain. To remove this, reset the machine to programme 3 – high flow, lower vacuum and low power.

If the epinucleus and cortex were adequately freed at the hydrodissection stage of the operation, increasing the AFR will drag this remaining, soft material to the mouth of the phaco probe. This movement (Fig. 3.37a, b) is further helped by the gentle, direct nudging of the epinucleus with the manipulator, sliding it along the capsule until it is caught in the high flow of the BSS.

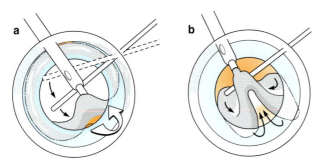

Fig. 3.37 Tackling the epinuclear shell

Phaco-chop (PC)

In eyes with very hard or bulky lenses, the use of the phaco-chopper as the manipulator is an excellent way of breaking up the nucleus into small fragments that will easily be removed with the phaco probe. It is a useful variation of the technique of nuclear fractis; in skilled hands the operation is quicker and less energy is needed to remove the nucleus.

The chopper has a long tip, which can easily get into the groove carved into the lens, even if this groove is quite short (Fig. 3.38). The lens can then be pulled apart with mechanical efficiency and minimal need for phaco power.

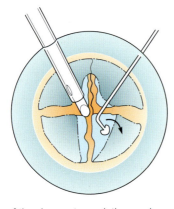

Fig. 3.38 Use of the chopper to crack the nucelus

TECHNIQUE

A central bowl is excavated and a single groove is sculpted. The nucleus is now cracked in half by the contrary movements of the chopper and phaco tip (Fig. 3.39a).

The lens is rotated through 90°. With the machine set in programme 2, the tip of the probe is buried into the middle of the half-nucleus – 'lolly-popping' the fragment (Fig. 3.39b), which is held by the high vacuum.

Pulling on the fragment creates a gap between nucleus and capsule, allowing the passage of the phaco-chopper over the equator of the lens. The chopper is then pulled back through the lens, towards the probe, cleaving the nucleus.

Repeated chopping manoeuvres will break the nucleus down into manageable fragments that are then emulsified. Individual fragments can be tackled in a similar way (Fig. 3.39c). The time taken and the total energy of phaco power needed is markedly reduced, but should not be undertaken by the inexperienced surgeon.

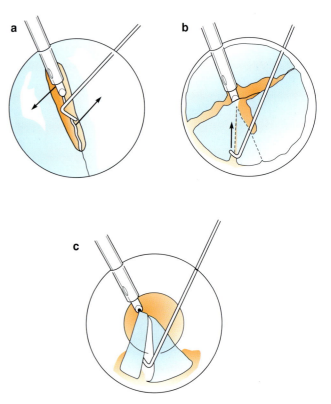

Fig. 3.39 The technique of 'phaco-chop'

CORTICAL TOILET AND CAPSULAR POLISHING

Although the epinucleus can be removed with the phaco probe in programme 3, soft epinucleus will also pass up the I/A port, especially if it is encouraged using the second instrument. This is a safer technique, especially for inexperienced surgeons.

The cortical layer may not be immediately obvious, but methodical searching will quickly reveal the cortical remnants in the fornices of the capsule. Search each quadrant of the capsule using the I/A probe. Start aspirating in the 12 o'clock position of the capsular fornix. It should be tackled first while it is splinted open by the remaining SLM (Fig. 3.40a).

The probe is moved slowly in a circular direction, keeping the port under the edge of the CCC. Initially, the SLM will occlude the port, and then, as the vacuum builds up, it will disappear up the probe. Use the (falling) vacuum at the tip to attract the next piece of cortex, and move the I/A steadily around the CCC margin in constant engagement with the SLM (Fig. 3.40b). Remove all visible fibres of SLM adherent to the capsule. The manipulator is useful to push, feed and free plugs of SLM and prevent the probe from clogging.

Having removed all visible cortical remnants, the interior of the anterior capsule is polished internally with the probe in order to reduce the capsular thickening.

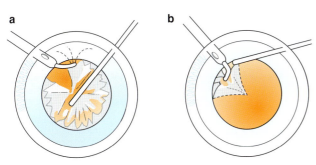

Fig 3.40 Aspirating cortical material

IOL implantation

Viscoelastic is injected and the incision enlarged to accommodate the chosen lens. Care must be taken to remain in the same plane as you enlarge the incision. Wounds tend to leak around their edges where the valve effect can be lost.

Each foldable and rigid lens has its own technique for insertion. Flexible silicone or acrylic IOLs can be folded or injected and introduced through small incisions of approx. 3.2 mm. Plate lenses made out of PMMA need larger incisions (approx. 5.5 mm), but if a scleral/phaco tunnel is used, suturing is not usually required.

Wound closure

Sutures must be used if the wound is not watertight resulting in collapse of the anterior chamber or if you are not sure whether it is watertight or not. Consider the patient, their activities and likelihood of complying with instructions postoperatively. Never be shy of using a stitch if unsure. They should be used when there is a risk of the

patient rubbing their eye, for instance if the patient is mentally handicapped. Scleral tunnels require suturing less often and because they are tunnelled into vascular tissue, they have the propensity to heal rapidly.

SUTURE TECHNIQUES

There are three suture patterns that can be used, e.g. 'box' suture, 'infinity' suture or radial interrupted. These sutures will close the wound and should not induce more astigmatism if placed carefully. (Remember that a wound which droops or sags will produce astigmatism against the rule, and of a type which is not as easily remedied as by removal of the suture at the appropriate time postoperatively.) Use either 10/0 nylon or 10/0 vicryl.

Box suture   The first bite of the suture runs along 75% of the length of the limbal edge of the wound (Fig. 3.41a). The needle is now passed through the cornea from the deep to superficial surface and at right-angles to the wound itself (Fig. 3.41b). Pass the needle through the corneal surface to the deep interface at its lateral extent (Fig. 3.41c). Tie the knot having reformed the eye with BSS and checked that the wound is now watertight (Fig. 3.41d). The suture ends are trimmed so that they lie buried in the wound.

Infinity suture   This is an alternative to a box suture and can be better for larger wounds. The first bite is oblique,

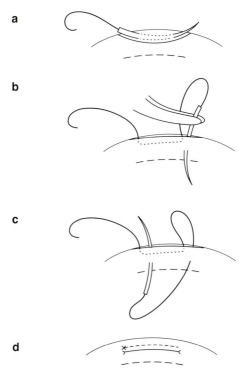

Fig. 3.41 Tying a 'box suture'

from the depth of the wound out onto the scleral surface (Fig. 3.42a), towards the surgeon. The second bite, which also takes an oblique course, passes through both cornea and sclera, crossing the first bite, approximately 3 mm lateral to the first (Fig. 3.42b). Now pass the needle through from corneal surface towards the crossing point of the suture, emerging out of the wound so that the knot can be tied deeply. The suture will now lie in the pattern of the mathematical sign of 'infinity' (∞) (Fig. 3.42c, d). Again, reform the eye with BSS, put on the first throws and recheck for leaks, reform again if necessary. The knot is completed.

Interrupted stitch   A single radial stitch (Fig. 3.43) is particularly useful for short wounds, such as a clear corneal incision. Drive the needle through both surfaces, but ensure that the needle picks up the floor of the tunnel as it passes through; the aim is to affix the lips of the wound front to back and not side to side. If the pull encourages the superficial faces to slide over the deep face the wound will distort, causing marked astigmatism.

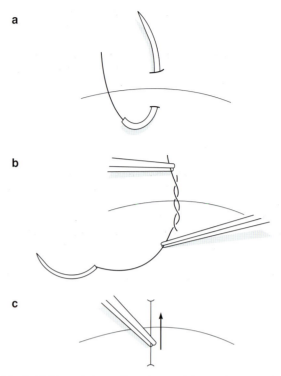

Fig. 3.43 The technique of inserting a radial stitch. Note that the needle passes radially but also along the length of the incision, preventing overriding by the superficial layer

CHALLENGING CASES

There are some cases that are more difficult and their management needs a thoughtful approach.

Small pupils

Pupils may not dilate well for a number of reasons, including pseudoexfoliation syndrome, previous iritis, diabetes or previous treatment with pilocarpine.

Encourage pupillary dilatation with the additional use of non-steroidal anti-inflammatory drops as a preoperative medication. The routine use of 1:1 000 000 adrenaline in the infusion helps dilatation in eyes that have not responded to routine drops; merely run the infusion through the eye for a few minutes without attempting any surgical advance on the cataract. This should work at any stage in the operation provided there is no mechanical factor stopping the pupil getting bigger.

However, where there are posterior synechiae or sphincter atrophy, a physical method must be used, e.g. sweeping and stretching the pupil margin with a fine cannula and injecting viscoelastic.

Multiple small sphincterotomies will divide the hyaline membrane that is sometimes seen but tends to leave iris strands that can be aspirated by the phaco tip. The pupil

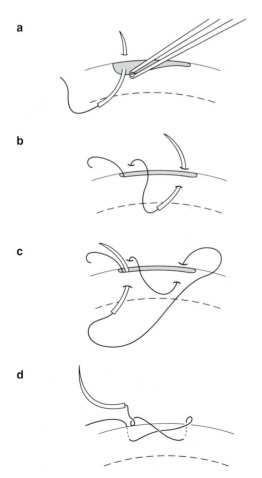

Fig. 3.42 Tying an 'infinity suture'

may be irregular postoperatively, but this is of a lesser consideration than not having any view of the lens when trying to remove it.

An elegant approach is the use of iris hooks. These are made of 6/0 prolene bent into a hook shape. They have a moveable flange that locks them in place.

PLACING IRIS HOOKS

Four equally spaced limbal stabs are made using an MVR blade, avoiding the sites for the main phaco incision and second instrument insertion (Fig. 3.44a).

Each hook is introduced horizontally through the incision and once in the anterior chamber is rotated so that the edge of the pupil is captured and pulled back towards the incision (Fig. 3.44b).

The shaft tip is grasped with a pair of suture-tying forceps whilst the plastic flange is slid up to the corneal surface, locking the hook at the external edge of the wound (Fig. 3.44c). The procedure is repeated for the remaining three hooks (Fig. 3.44d). If the lens is unstable, the iris hooks can be repositioned to pass around the capsulorrhexis to protect against dislocation (Fig. 3.44e).

To remove the hooks, gently ease the flange, disengage the iris margin and rapidly pull the hooks through the corneal wound (Fig. 3.44f).

Alternatively, the pupil can be stretched using two hooks (Fig. 3.45) or by using a proprietary pupil stretcher (Fig. 3.46). Both these methods will rupture the tissues at the pupil margin and leave the pupil atonic (it was probably already so).

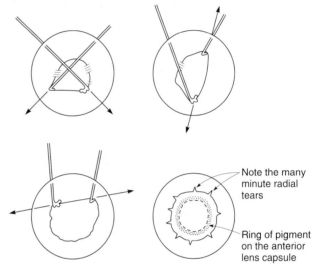

Note the many minute radial tears

Ring of pigment on the anterior lens capsule

Fig. 3.45 Using two hooks to stretch the pupil

White cataract

The difficulties with these types of cataract are in visualizing the CCC and dealing with the milky liquid which usually floods into the anterior chamber as soon as the capsule is pierced. Without a red reflex, tearing the CCC is very difficult, but if the AC is irrigated thoroughly a better view can sometimes be obtained and the CCC started. The use of a light pipe, with the room lights out, can help visualize the structures.

Staining the capsule with trypan blue is the easiest option. Air is first injected, displacing the aqueous, then 1 ml of trypan blue (Visionblue) is injected and left in the anterior chamber for one minute. BSS is then used to wash the dye out of the eye (two or three 2 ml syringes may be needed). After injecting viscoelastic, the CCC is then started. Use the I/A probe to aspirate any 'lens milk', irrigating until the view clears. The blue capsule is now easily seen against the white background of the lens; the CCC is completed in the normal way.

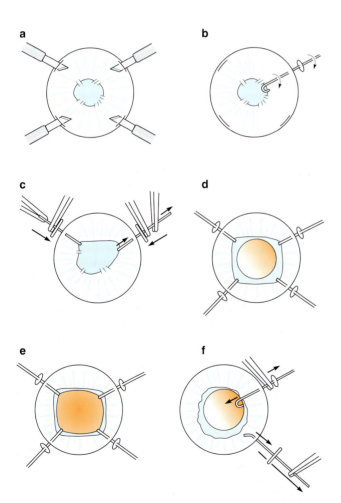

a

b

c

d

e

f

Fig. 3.44 The use of iris hooks for pupillary dilatation and lens stabilization

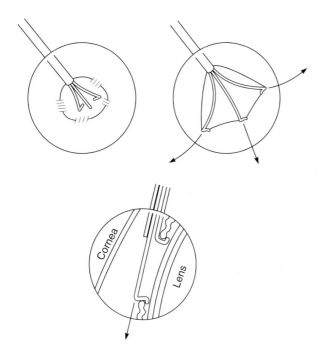

Fig. 3.46 The use of a pupil-stretcher

Preoperative lens instability

Frank irido- or phacodenesis suggests zonular weakness. In cases of pseudoexfoliation syndrome, zonular weakness is common even in the absence of frank lens instability. In these cases anticipate problems by inserting a capsule tension ring after hydrodissection. The ring can be injected into the capsule with a patent introducer but it is as easy to feed the ring into the capsule manually. The topic of zonular weakness and techniques to deal with this are discussed in the next chapter.

Preoperative astigmatism

The placing of the incisions for phacoemulsification can affect the astigmatism of a patient's cornea. This can be used strategically to reduce the cylindrical correction. Astigmatism can be reduced by making the phaco incision at the end of the axis of the positive cylinder. For example, if the patient has astigmatism preoperatively of +2.00 cyl @ 90°, the cylinder will tend to be reduced if placed around the 12 o'clock meridian.

Similarly, the cylindrical error can be increased by making the incision at 90° to the plus cylinder; for example, if a patient has a preoperative cylinder of +2.00 cyl @ 180°, their astigmatism will tend to be increased if the phaco incision is based around the 12 o'clock meridian. If the incision is corneal, and enlarged to take the IOL and then not sutured, the sag in the cornea will aggravate the problem even further.

The effect can be enhanced by making concentric keratotomies in the diametrically opposite cornea. The effects of this surgery can be unpredictable and where there is any doubt, refractive surgery should be performed as a separate, secondary procedure. This topic is beyond the scope of this book and needs specific study.

Endothelial degeneration

The trauma of cataract surgery can lead to corneal decompensation in eyes that have compromised endothelial function, for example Fuch's endothelial dystrophy. The prophylactic use of a viscoelastic that will stay in the anterior chamber during surgery will protect the endothelium. The theory is that the viscoelastic molecules are shorter and not cohesively linked with each other; as a result, the ebb and flow in the anterior chamber will not readily suck them out of the eye during surgery and the viscoelastic will remain in place to protect the endothelium. In practice, at the end of the phaco phase some will still be found in the eye. Manufacturers recommend agents such as Viscoat, Amvisc, Healonid 5 for these properties; they each have their own protractors and detractors but on the whole work reasonably well.

Remember that if this sort of 'non-cohesive' viscoelastic is used to help during lens implantation, it must be deliberately removed at the end of the operation or a considerable rise in IOP will follow postoperatively. On the whole it is better to use a different, 'cohesive' viscoelastic for lens implantation because it is much more easily removed after the IOL is in place. Budgetary constraints may prevent the luxury of two agents for one eye!

Preoperative uveitis

Pre-existing uveitis may be exacerbated or reactivated by surgery. Surgery should not be done if there is active inflammation present. Pre-treat the eye until quiet. Administer an IV bolus of methyl prednisolone (250–500 mg) when the patient arrives in the operating theatre.

Part Two

Managing Surgical Difficulties and Complications

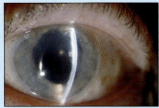

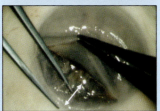

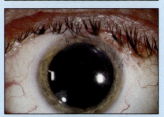

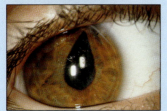

Surgical complications and their management

INTRODUCTION

In ECCE, even though quite serious complications can occur, it is usually possible to deal with the problem and then return to complete the planned operation. The technique has a greater range of tolerance than phaco. Capsular problems, for instance, which may require abandonment or conversion of phaco, can be handled adroitly because the eye is already open and the section will, in any case, need to be sutured.

In phaco, each step of the operation is important to the next. If a problem occurs early on this will directly predicate against the subsequent manoeuvres, each of which relies on successfully completing earlier ones. This game of consequences makes the compelling argument for mastering each and every stage of phaco. It is also the reason why when teaching or learning phaco, the trainees should start with the last steps and learn them in reverse order, finishing with the incision. If a problem occurs towards the end of the operation there are fewer steps that might be affected.

The problems that complicate each of the steps of phaco surgery are discussed in turn. Minor complications managed successfully will allow you to continue with the planned surgery but major complications will mean abandoning phaco and converting to ECCE or some other form of salvage procedure.

INCISION PHASE

Problems with incisions

It is hoped when using small incision techniques that the surgical incisions will be watertight without the need for suturing and that astigmatic change will be neutral. Wounds that are too large or poorly constructed have a tendency to leak and will often require suturing. Wounds

that are too small will be distorted by the phaco probe or IOL as they are forced through.

If the 'corneal' stab wound is made too far posteriorly, the conjunctiva at the limbus may be opened and the irrigating fluid will have a tendency to inflate the conjunctiva. This rapidly enlarging bleb obscures the view of the superior cornea. To decompress this collection, two generous radial cuts can be made into this billowing conjunctiva about 5 mm behind the limbus with spring scissors.

Any surgical wound of the eye should be watertight at the end of the operation. If not safely closed, bacterial contamination readily occurs. If you are anxious about the integrity of the section, do not hesitate to suture the wound. Suturing should also be considered for any patient who is very frail or who lives alone, especially with co-existing blepharitis or when compliance is a potential problem.

Descemet's membrane separation (DMS)

Localized, limited stripping of Descemet's membrane with attached endothelium frequently occurs. Minor degrees of separation around the internal mouth of the incisions develop during the passage in and out of the instruments (Fig. 4.1). Snagging of this membrane is aggravated by the infusion sleeve and the irrigating fluid which causes its extension. Using a blunt keratome to make the incision or entering the eye at a very oblique angle are other causes. Separation will usually be seen as instruments and the IOL are introduced into the eye and particular care must be taken to prevent this extending.

A decision about whether or not to deal with the problem can be made at the end of the operation. Minor degrees of separation around the incision can be left and are of no clinical significance. When involving more than a fifth of the area of the cornea, the lesion cannot be left. Something must be done or the cornea will decompensate

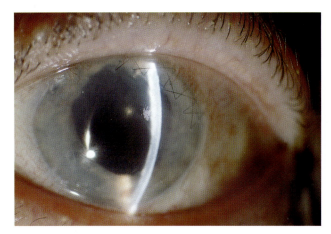

Fig. 4.1 Corneal thickening as a result of localized separation of Descemet's membrane

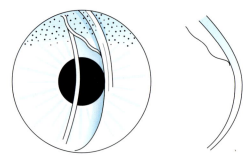

Fig. 4.2 Descemet's membrane separation

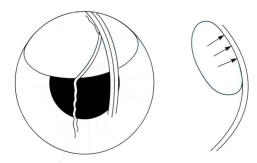

Fig. 4.3 Treatment of Descemet's membrane separation with an expansile gas bubble

as fluid is forced between the stromal lamellae (Fig. 4.1). The management of choice is to inject a bubble of an expansile gas (SF$_6$) which will tamponade the separated membrane back in place (Box 4.1; Figs 4.2 and 4.3).

An alternative approach is direct suturing. The anterior chamber is filled with viscoelastic and using 10/0 nylon the wound is sutured through and through, including Descemet's membrane. A mattress suture is best in these circumstances (Fig. 4.4). Even with an eye completely filled with viscoelastic, it can still be difficult to get the membrane neatly held by the suture.

The patient should be closely monitored and specialist advice sought if the cornea does not settle.

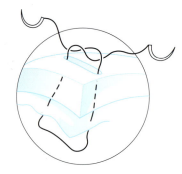

Fig. 4.4 Suturing a Descemet's membrane separation back into place

CAPSULE

Continuous curvilinear capsulorrhexis (CCC)

STRENGTH OF CCC

The strength and elasticity of a CCC allow remarkable control of intraocular manipulation, and when its creation goes astray the safe completion of the whole operation is put at risk. A CCC is normally fashioned by careful tearing but may also be made using an intraocular capsular diathermy. The strength of the *torn* CCC has been shown to be stronger than one made with the capsular diathermy due to its smooth edge (Fig. 4.5). When the diathermy-cut CCC is

---

Box 4.1 Injecting SF$_6$ to replace separated Descemet's membrane

▶ Attach a sterile air filter to a 5 ml syringe

▶ Draw up 2.5 ml of SF$_6$ gas followed by 2.5 ml of air

▶ Using a Rycroft cannula, inject a bubble of gas through the opposite port to that which has the DMS

▶ The anterior chamber should be half-filled thus rolling the flap of Descemet's membrane back into place

▶ Posture the patient so that the bubble pushes against the dehiscence (if a temporal incision was used, the patient will need to posture on the opposite cheek)

▶ The bubble should persist for 10 days ensuring re-adhesion

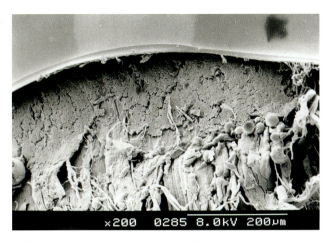

Fig. 4.5 Electronmicrograph of a torn CCC

examined on scanning electron microscopy it is seen to have a jagged edge with multiple radial micro-tears (Fig. 4.6). This explains the relative weakness and increased likelihood of radial tears using the diathermy technique.

As the surgeon starts the CCC there is usually satisfactory progress. Once the 6 o'clock position is reached and the tear is recurved towards the 12 o'clock position, there is a tendency for the CCC to begin to stray towards the periphery. If the leading edge of the rhexis disappears behind the iris the tear can extend to the equator and around to the posterior capsule (PC). Serious complications, such as loss of nucleus, threaten.

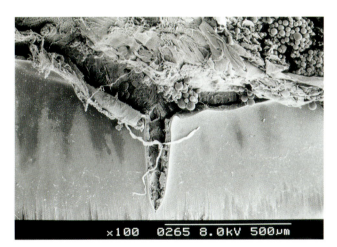

Fig. 4.6 Electronmicrograph of a CCC created with capsular diathermy

SIZE OF CCC

If the CCC is too large, the nucleus will tend to herniate into the anterior chamber during hydrodissection. The lens should be balloted back into place using the hydrodissection cannula. Postoperatively, the large CCC will let the

optic pass through into the posterior chamber which will allow the anterior and posterior capsules to fibrose together. When this happens, the IOL may become displaced away from the visual axis, producing edge effects such as glare and haloes disturbing an otherwise technically satisfactory result.

Tearing a CCC in a child or adolescent is different from in an adult. In a child the capsule is considerably more elastic and less easy to control. For this reason, it is better to aim for a smaller CCC initially which can be enlarged later in the operation.

If the CCC is too small, removing the peripheral cortex can be difficult and clumsy manipulations may tear the capsule. The long-term problems of fibrosis of the capsular rim can cause shrinkage of this opening (phimosis) which can reduce vision and require treatment (Fig. 4.7). If this happens, the anterior capsule can be opened by Nd-YAG laser (Fig. 4.8).

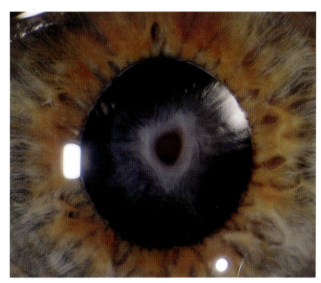

Fig. 4.7 Capsular phimosis pre-laser

MANAGEMENT OF A 'LOST' CCC

There are a number of options to manage and control a CCC which is extending towards the equator (Fig. 4.9a). Most importantly, you should stop tearing and refill the eye with viscoelastic. This will relieve the tension on the zonules and make it easier to control the tear.

Using Utratas forceps the very apex of the tear is pulled gently towards the centre of the pupil until the tear's direction is changed (Fig. 4.9b). This results in a small notch in the CCC which is a potential weakness (Fig. 4.9c).

If this does not work or looks too frightening, you should return to where you started the CCC. If there is a tag of capsule you can start to tear another CCC in the opposite direction in a route that will bring you back to the point at which you abandoned previously. You may

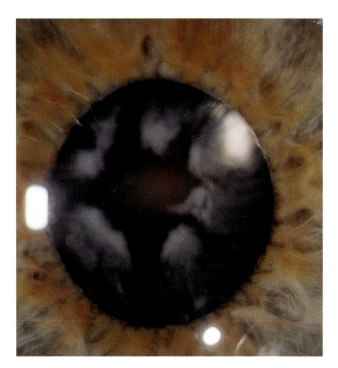

Fig. 4.8 Capsular phimosis post-laser

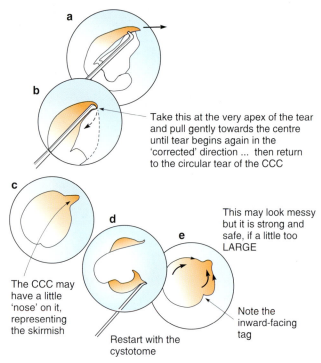

Take this at the very apex of the tear and pull gently towards the centre until tear begins again in the 'corrected' direction ... then return to the circular tear of the CCC

The CCC may have a little 'nose' on it, representing the skirmish

Restart with the cystotome

This may look messy but it is strong and safe, if a little too LARGE

Note the inward-facing tag

Fig. 4.9 (a) A CCC tear heading towards the equator; **(b)** redirecting a peripheral CCC with forceps; **(c,d,e)** restarting the CCC

need to use the cystotome or scissors to create a tag to hold onto (Fig. 4.9d, e).

With care and luck it may be possible to avert the danger and keep a continuous torn edge to the CCC. If the capsulotomy was only achieved by using either capsular diathermy or with an irregular restart of the tear at another position, the CCC will no longer be continuous (Fig. 4.10a, b). The loss of elastic strength threatens an unexpected radial tear which can later extend, leading to loss of nuclear fragments into the posterior segment. The capsule should therefore be treated as if it already has a small radial tear (see later in this section). If the patient has a large or hard lens, it may be better to convert to an ECCE technique, particularly when the surgeon is inexperienced.

If a decision is made to convert, the control and strength of the CCC is no longer required and a wide opening is needed through which the lens can be extruded. The capsule opening is opened using Long Ong's scissors which creates episiotomies that are crucial to allow the nucleus to be expressed (Fig. 4.11). If the capsule opening is not big enough for the lens, the capsule may rupture or vitreous will herniate round.

ZONULAR WEAKNESS (ZW)

Zonular weakness reduces the radial tension on the capsule. This makes it harder to tear the CCC. Zonular weakness may be essential (EZW) or acquired (AZW). The latter is usually the result of trauma or extended surgical manoeuvres which shear the zonule fibres.

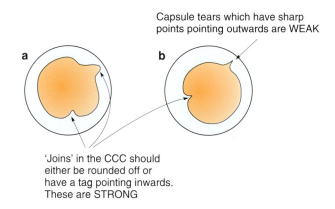

Capsule tears which have sharp points pointing outwards are WEAK

'Joins' in the CCC should either be rounded off or have a tag pointing inwards. These are STRONG

Fig 4.10 Outward pointing notches in the CCC are potential weak areas

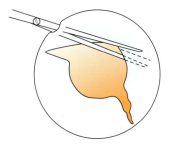

Fig. 4.11 Opening the capsule with Long Ong's scissors

ZW may be anticipated preoperatively when there is a history of blunt trauma or where there are signs of pseudoexfoliation or phacodenesis (Box 4.2; Figs 4.12–4.15).

Box 4.2 Causes of zonular weakness

ESSENTIAL

▶ Iris/lens coloboma
▶ Marfan's/homocysteinuria
▶ Pseudoexfoliation syndrome (PES)
▶ Very elderly
▶ Hypermature cataracts

ACQUIRED

▶ History of lens/blunt eye trauma
▶ Surgical trauma

Sometimes ZW is found unexpectedly as the surgeon begins to do the CCC. The early signs of potential problems may be subtle. As the viscoelastic is injected the lens–iris diaphragm settles a long way back. Phaco- or iridodenesis may be seen. As the CCC starts, the capsule will bunch up. Traction on the leading edge may cause the whole lens to move from side to side precluding progress of the CCC. With this gross movement, insertion of a capsule tension ring (CTR) will be of little benefit and you should convert to an intracapsular extraction of the lens. If there has been a posterior tear in the capsule, traction with the cryoprobe may end up removing the capsule, allowing the nucleus to slip backwards and remain in the eye (Figs 4.16 and 4.17). In this situation, the nucleus may need to be retrieved in the same way as for dropped fragments during phaco (see later).

With EZW the surgeon must anticipate problems. The CCC should be small and central. Hydrodissection and/or delineation should be as complete as possible before any intralenticular manoeuvres are started which can cause further damage to the zonule. Nucleus manipulations must be gentle and smooth. Folds may appear and some

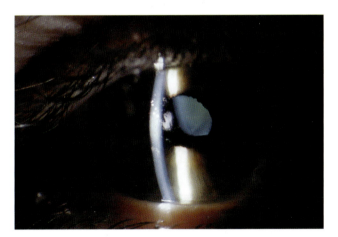

Fig. 4.12 Marfan's syndrome

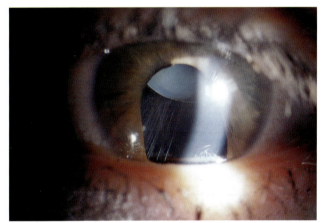

Fig. 4.14 Coloboma (exfoliative)

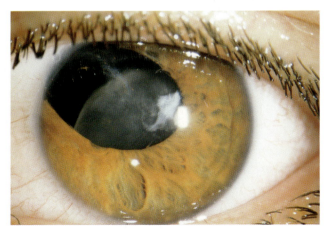

Fig. 4.13 Post-traumatic zonular weakness

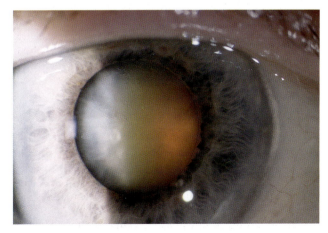

Fig. 4.15 Pseudoexfoliation

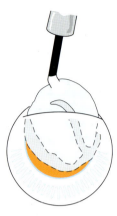

Fig. 4.16 Cryoextraction of the capsule without the lens when there is a pre-existing posterior capsular tear

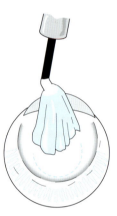

Fig. 4.17 Cryoextraction of the capsule

arcs may be impossible to tear. Implantation of a capsule tension ring (CTR) at this early stage should allow you to complete the CCC. If it is impossible to penetrate the capsule and the lens wobbles wildly from side to side, it is unwise to persist and safer to proceed to intracapsular surgery (see above).

IRIS

Just as a perfectly torn CCC is the most robust aperture in the anterior capsule, so does a fully dilated and healthy iris contribute to the visualization of the lens during surgery.

Direct phaco tip damage to the iris usually occurs as the tip is brought up at the end of a grooving sweep (Fig. 4.18). For a right-handed surgeon this will be in the 4 o'clock position. Any damaged iris tends to be repeatedly aspirated into the phaco tip, further compounding the problem. You should try to keep the phaco tip deeper in the anterior chamber and to use the anterior cortex to shield vacuum from the iris strands.

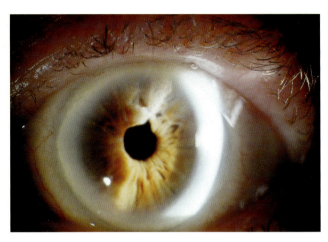

Fig. 4.18 Iris damage by phaco tip

PHACOEMULSIFICATION PHASE

The need for coordination of all four limbs and the presence of a very sharp, potentially destructive instrument in the anterior chamber make the phaco phase the most daunting for new or inexperienced surgeons. Subtle alterations to the normal progress of the surgery may represent the start of a more serious complication. Recognition of these abnormal changes is crucial to minimize the effects (see Table 4.1).

The following complications will be dealt with in greater detail:

1 radial tear
2 PC hole
3 posterior loss of nuclear material
4 zonular dehiscence.

Radial tear

A radial tear is an important complication and in certain circumstances it is foolhardy to proceed. Even a small tear means that the CCC has lost its integrity. The tear may extend posteriorly as the manipulations of phaco continue, creating a gap that nuclear fragments can fall backwards through. Alternatively, vitreous can suddenly present, preventing easy removal of remaining fragments or cortical material.

If a small tear is noticed at the end of the phaco phase, cortical toilet and lens implantation may be safely completed without further remark. However, when a radial tear is spotted before commencing phaco, great care and experience will be required if the surgeon is to proceed and safely complete the planned operation. If the tear seems to be extending it is safer to convert than to continue. There

Table 4.1 Complications during phacoemulsification phase

Observation	Adverse event	Threatened
Radial tear	Radial tear	Dramatic extension
Unable to rotate nucleus	Incomplete hydrodissection	Zonular damage
Sudden deepening of a/c	PC rupture/zonular dehiscence	Dropped nucleus
Failure of aspiration	PC hole and vitreous presentation	Vitreous traction
Lens instability	Zonular rupture	Lens dislocation
Sudden shallowing and iris prolapse	Suprachoroidal haemorrhage	Expulsive haemorrhage

are a number of other circumstances where conversion to large incision ECCE-type surgery is indicated (Table 4.2).

If it is felt safe to continue with phacoemulsification, great care must be taken to minimize manipulations which put torsional and anteroposterior forces on the capsule because they can encourage posterior extension of any tear (Box 4.3). (See Figs 4.19 and 4.20.)

If the tear has obviously extended posteriorly, phacoemulsification should be abandoned. Conversion to the ECCE technique will allow more controlled removal of

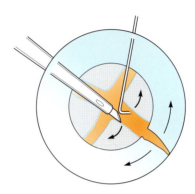

Fig. 4.19 Cracking the nucleus in the same meridian as a tear will encourage its extension

Table 4.2 Relative contraindications to proceeding with phaco in the presence of a radial tear

Condition	Reason
Small pupil	No view
Young eye	Springy zonule
High myopia	Vitreous pressure, scleral collapse
Hard lens	Extended surgery
Restless patient	Unpredictable control
Pseudoexfoliation syndrome	Further complicating factor
Large lens	Risk of further extension of the tear

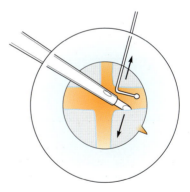

Fig. 4.20 Nuclear fractis in another meridian is safer

the nucleus (Box 4.4). The corneal wound must be enlarged, the capsulorrhexis opened and the nucleus removed, if possible, in one piece. The use of an irrigating vectis to deliver the lens prevents an excessive rise in vitreous pressure so keeping its anterior prolapse to a minimum. Unless the surgeon is very lucky, an anterior vitrectomy is usually required (Fig. 4.21).

Posterior capsule hole

Any hole or tear in the posterior capsule threatens prolapse of vitreous with a cascade of problems. Some of these will

Box 4.3 Continuing phaco in the presence of a radial tear

▶ Completely free the nucleus by hydrodelineation within the cortical shell
▶ Do not hydrodissect the outer shell
▶ Emulsify nucleus inside protective envelope of SLM and cortex
▶ Minimize phaco time by increasing phaco power
▶ Ensure full-depth groove of nucleus before splitting
▶ Minimize manipulations and avoid putting stretching forces onto the capsule
▶ Crack the nucleus in a meridian away from the radial tear

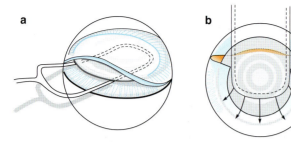

Fig. 4.21 Use of the irrigating vectis to remove the nucleus. The vectis is passed gently into the capsule, behind the nucleus and gently lifted. The nucleus should spontaneously move towards the exterior of the eye as the pressure of the infusion takes effect. Great care is needed not to cause further damage to the capsule

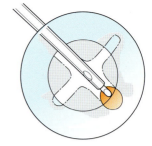

Fig. 4.22 A capsule hole is often found at the end of the groove, where the probe has passed right through the nucleus, cortex and capsule

---

Box 4.4 Conversion in the presence of a radial tear

▶ Enlarge the corneal wound to approximately 120°

▶ Open the capsulorrhexis with Ong's scissors, cutting out toward the equator of the capsule

▶ Elevate the upper pole of the lens nucleus by the injection and insinuation of viscoelastic behind it

▶ Introduce an irrigating vectis behind the lens

▶ Advance the vectis until the whole nucleus is supported

▶ Gently float the lens out of the eye

▶ Look for evidence for the presence of vitreous in the anterior chamber (an anterior vitrectomy will usually be needed)

▶ With either the I/A handpiece or vitrector, clean and aspirate any remaining cortical matter in the capsule

▶ Leave the anterior capsule alone; it will provide the platform for the sulcus fixation of the IOL

---

be immediate, such as difficulty in removing residual lens material, and some more remote, e.g. retinal detachment.

A hole may occur at any stage during the phaco phase but is usually noted as the first quadrant is removed (Box 4.5). The hole tends to be small and round and is usually found at the inferior extent of the axis taken by the tip of the phaco probe (for right-handed surgeons this will be at 4–5 o'clock, and at 7–8 o'clock for left-handers). It is usually caused by the phaco needle passing through the nucleus and its surrounding cortical shell (Fig. 4.22).

Once a hole is noticed, it is crucial to keep the instruments in the eye and to avoid rapid changes in intraocular pressure. This pressure will force the vitreous through the hole and out of the eye. Lower the intraocular pressure by reducing the height of the infusion bottle and stop all intraocular currents by stopping the infusion and aspiration. (Vitreous is a slow moving substance except when hydrated or when the infusion pressure is suddenly released and there is an exit by which to leave.) It follows that if the probe is taken out of the eye when under the added pressure of the infusion, the vitreous will move directly to the incision ports and span the operative field. The infusion bottle must be lowered to reduce the IOP and prevent the vortex of current which will hydrate the vitreous and encourage its prolapse. If the bottle is high, re-entry by the phaco probe will cause distension of the capsular bag, which in turn will extend the hole, causing additional vitreous migration.

A moment should be taken to assess the situation and think what opportunities are afforded. The surgeon should consider converting to extracapsular extraction.

If the cortical shell is otherwise intact, and has been freed so that it is able to move independently (by previous, adequate hydrodelineation and hydrodissection), it may be rotated to cover the hole (Fig. 4.23a–c). The injection of a dispersive viscoelastic to cover the posterior capsular rent can tamponade the hole allowing clearance of residual lens material. Cohesive viscoelastics will tend to be aspirated easily into the phaco probe, making it unsuitable to plug a capsular defect.

Nuclear fragments can be controlled with the second instrument, keeping them away from the capsular hole. It is important to ensure that aspiration and vacuum are only applied when the phaco tip is nuzzled into cortical and lens fragments. By these quick manipulations it may be possible to complete the phacoemulsification without further agitation of the anterior vitreous face or loss of fragments into the vitreous.

After the nuclear fragments have been removed aspiration of the remaining cortical shell should be possible without drawing the vitreous forward. The flow and the bottle should be low and the I/A cannula directed into the cortex and away from the hole. Aspiration close to the hole will pull vitreous forward into the anterior segment. Once prolapsed it will become intertwined with the cortical and capsular tissues and an anterior vitrectomy becomes obligatory.

If a posterior capsular hole is noticed towards the end of the phaco phase or during irrigation/aspiration, it may be

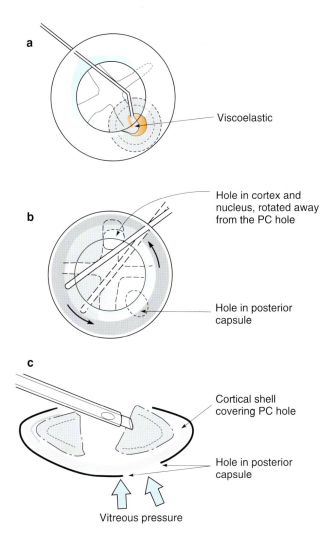

Fig. 4.23 The cortical shell is dialled around to cover the capsular hole

Vitreous loss and management of remaining nucleus

'I never lose vitreous – I always know where I've put it!'
(Anon.)

Sudden presentation of vitreous into the operative field during the phaco phase of the operation is a major complication which requires a clear and strategic approach. The threat of loss of lens material into the posterior segment heralds a stormy course unless managed carefully. Depending on the amount of nuclear material that remains when vitreous is first noted, the management of the lens will be different and ancillary manoeuvres will be required. In any case an anterior vitrectomy will be required.

possible to convert it to a posterior CCC (Fig. 4.24). A torn circular gap has the same inherent strength as that performed in the anterior capsule thus preventing enlargement of the defect. This is especially important when the time comes to implant the IOL.

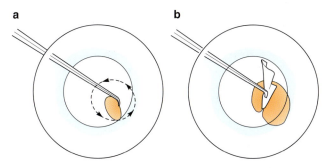

Fig. 4.24 A posterior CCC can be torn to make the posterior capsular hole stronger, limiting its ability to extend further

Posterior passage of nuclear material through the posterior capsule

WHOLE NUCLEUS

Loss of the nucleus or fragments of the lens may occur rapidly. Large PC rents usually follow extension of a radial tear or of a small posterior capsular hole made earlier. During the process of nuclear cracking or during prolonged manipulation of a hard nucleus these rips can dramatically increase. In eyes that have developed a cataract following trauma, the surgeon should be wary of a 'silent' hole in the posterior capsule which can extend during hydrodissection

The first suggestion of a problem is often a sudden deepening of the anterior chamber. The nucleus will then be seen to pitch and move posteriorly. Because of its shape, the surgeon will find the nucleus difficult to grasp to prevent its further posterior passage. A dash to grab the nucleus with forceps must be resisted.

In theory, there are two options to try to prevent a nucleus from disappearing posteriorly through a hole in the capsule:

1 The nucleus can be speared with the rapid insertion of a 21G needle through the paracentesis incision or pars plana (Fig. 4.25). Once the lens has been transfixed, the section is enlarged to 7–9 mm, depending on nuclear size. Heavy or regular viscoelastic may be useful to help manipulate lens fragments. The section should be large enough to either express, float or remove the nucleus with an irrigating vectis. (The insertion of a 21G needle carries a risk of damaging the CCC or, if passed through the pars plana, the ciliary body, iris or retina.)

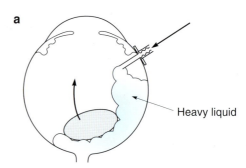

Heavy liquid

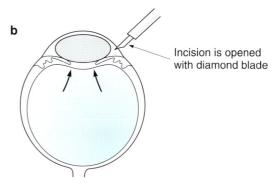

Incision is opened with diamond blade

Fig. 4.27 Use of heavy liquid to float lens off the retina

immediately. If not, it is better to close the eye and refer the patient to a vitreo-retinal colleague who will be better able to complete the surgery (Fig. 4.27).

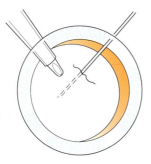

Fig. 4.25 Spearing lens nucleus with 21 gauge needle

2 The surgeon can let the nucleus go. In practice when the nucleus drops it happens quickly and often before any sort of surgical response can be attempted. The temptation to chase the nucleus with phaco probe, cryo-probe or forceps should be resisted because there are significant risks of damaging the eye. (Traction on the vitreous base, retinal tears, retinal detachment or vitreous haemorrhage.) Arrangements must then be made to later remove the lens. If experienced with vitreo-retinal techniques and the use of heavy liquid, the surgeon may elect to proceed to this

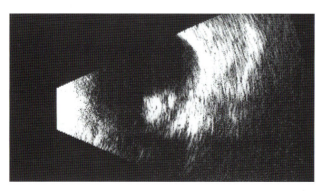

Fig. 4.26 Ultrasonogram of lens lying on the retina

Box 4.6 Actions to handle threatened loss of nuclear material

▶ **Stop** aspirating, but stay in the eye
▶ **Drop the bottle height** to lower intraocular pressure
▶ Pass the manipulator or any fine cannula behind the nucleus to stop it falling backwards
▶ Place heavy viscoelastic behind the lens to support it (unlikely to work)
▶ Try to spear the lens with 21G needle if nucleus seems to be falling
▶ Assess
▶ **Convert** – open the incision to 10 mm
▶ Open the CCC with episiotomies
▶ Encourage the lens into the anterior chamber with a dialling hook
▶ Deliver the lens with an irrigating vectis
▶ Anterior vitrectomy

Loss of nucleus or fragments carries the risk of an aggressive uveitis or secondary glaucoma developing if not managed properly. Postoperatively the patient will have to be treated with intensive topical steroids and probably acetazolamide if the IOP begins to rise.

NUCLEAR FRAGMENTS

A PC hole may be difficult to see, even if two of the four quadrants have already been removed. A subtle clue to the presence of a hole may be the inability to gain an aspirating 'hold' on a piece of nucleus. This is because the aspiration port is clogged with vitreous. Once a PC rupture is suspected or a hole is found it is important to keep control of the fluid dynamics of the anterior chamber. Instruments should be left in the eye, and the height of the infusion bottle reduced to about 20 cm above the eye. The intraocular forces will reduce and the rate of events will slow down. As the infusion pressure falls off, the phaco probe can be removed from the eye and lens matter and vitreous will no longer leap for the incision port. The lens fragments are now best removed with a vitreous cutter or through an extended section as for extracapsular surgery.

Small fragments, less than a quarter of the nucleus, that are lost posteriorly may be left and treated conservatively. Although secondary uveitis and glaucoma frequently develop, these can usually be managed with medical treatment alone until the material is resorbed. Larger fragments will need removal as discussed above, but early discussions with a vitreo-retinal colleague are useful in recruiting their timely help if problems develop.

If the remaining nuclear fragments are left contained in the capsular bag, the first procedure required is an anterior vitrectomy, with care being taken to corral the fragments in the bag and later remove these with the vitreous cutter (Fig. 4.28a–d) (see also Box 4.7).

Postoperatively, care must be taken to watch for a rise in IOP and inflammation. If this occurs, appropriate treatment with anti-hypertensives and the frequent application of steroids will be required and surgical removal must be considered. In any eye in which nuclear fragments may possibly have been lost into the posterior segment (i.e. any eye with a large capsular tear/rent), the posterior segment should be examined in the days following surgery. A late, sterile endophthalmitis may be the first clue that such fragments have fallen backwards.

It is crucial that the anterior chamber is free of vitreous before proceeding to lens implantation. Sweeping a Rycroft cannula across the internal incision apertures will free any vitreous threads from the wounds. Movement of instruments inside an anterior chamber containing vitreous will lead to distortion of the remaining capsular elements (see Fig. 4.28d).

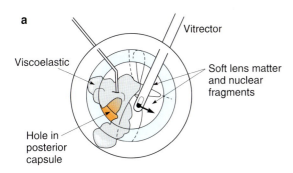

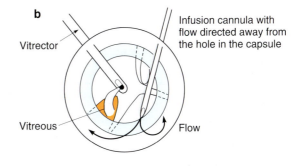

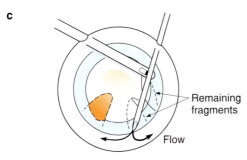

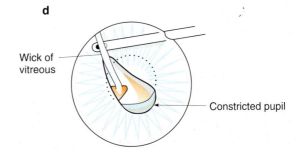

Fig. 4.28 Anterior vitrectomy with fragments

Box 4.7 Performing an anterior vitrectomy in the presence of lens fragments

▶ Tell the nursing staff to prepare the vitrector – this takes time

▶ Lower the bottle height to equilibrate intraocular pressure

▶ Using the manipulator, prevent the fragments tumbling backwards

▶ Remove the phaco probe and re-inflate the eye with viscoelastic (some authorities advise the use of 'heavy' viscoelastic such as Healonid GV)

▶ Remove the second instrument once the fragments are barricaded with viscoelastic

▶ Enlarge the second incision, angling the knife towards the inner opening of the phaco stab. (This will give easier access to lens fragments and vitreous)

▶ Introduce an infusion cannula into the second incision (e.g. Butterfly 19G IV cannula) directing the flow over the iris surface and *away* from the capsular hole and not into the vitreous which would encourage further presentation

▶ Remove the lens fragments as they present to the cutter. Occlude the port of the cutter with lens remnants and hold them there by the increased vacuum at the tip

▶ Use the distal end of the infusion cannula to feed lens matter into the port and encourage its removal by this masticatory process. If the lens matter is either soft or mostly cortical there should be no difficulty

▶ Pass the cutter through the rent in the capsule and into the anterior vitreous. Using a cutting speed of approximately 360 cuts per minute, draw the vitreous from the anterior chamber posteriorly

▶ If the nucleus was already fractured and all the pieces remain, they will prove difficult to control. It is likely that one or more quadrants will be lost into the posterior segment. Do not chase them; some may come forward into the cutter or anterior chamber as the vitrectomy proceeds. If the pieces are very hard or bulky, the wounds may need to be enlarged

▶ The vitrectomy should continue until the anterior segment is clear of vitreous

▶ The CCC should be left untouched. It will later provide the means of securing a sulcus-fixated IOL

▶ Once the anterior segment is clear of vitreous, the incision is opened to allow the implantation of an IOL

Anterior vitrectomy

Conversion moves from an elective planned procedure to a salvage strategy if surgical complications have led to the prolapse of vitreous into the anterior chamber. An anterior vitrectomy will be required whenever vitreous presents. The procedure will also allow the safe removal of vitreous, lens fragments and cortex and divides connections between the anterior segment structures and the retina. Failure to understand why this is necessary and what happens if not done adequately is to underestimate the long-term pathological consequences of vitreous incarceration, which include cystoid macular oedema, retinal detachment and chronic uveitis.

The technique of anterior vitrectomy is a fundamental skill for any ophthalmic surgeon. If the surgeon feels comfortable with the method and its purpose, then the complication of capsule rupture and vitreous loss will always be competently handled. Familiarity in the use and setting up of vitreous cutting machinery is mandatory. Both surgical and theatre support staff must be able to play their part promptly if and when a vitrectomy is required in the anterior segment.

A vitreous cutter is essential to avoid retinal traction and to complete the toilet of the anterior segment It is danger-ous merely to swab the surgical wound with sponges and cut away the presenting vitreous strands with scissors. The end result of this is to leave vitreous incarcerated.

When a tear in the posterior capsule is noted or vitreous presents, the surgeon should stop operating and think. Instruments should not be taken out of the eye until the intraocular pressure has been reduced by lowering the bottle height. Nursing staff should be asked to prepare the vitrector – this takes time.

PREFERRED ANTERIOR VITRECTOMY TECHNIQUE (Figs 4.29–4.31)

1 Reinflate the eye using viscoelastic (heavy or normal).

2 Enlarge the second incision by half a diamond-blade's width, angling it to face the inner opening of the principal phaco incision. This will give a wider arc for the vitrector. It will afford an opportunity to remove any last strands of vitreous from the wound at the end of the operation.

3 Pass the vitrector through the rent in the capsule into the anterior vitreous (Fig. 4.29a).

4 Begin cutting (≥360 cuts per minute), drawing the vitreous in the anterior chamber posteriorly.

Worked Example 4.1

A 76-year-old female patient with past history of herpes simplex keratitis 23 years previously.

R eye previous, routine extracapsular cataract surgery with IOL implant. VA postoperatively was 6/9, refraction −0.50/ +0.50 × 10.

April 1999 Left phaco surgery: a very hard nucleus was found which was sculpted and cracked. A hard posterior shield linked the four fragments together preventing ready removal of the fragments. During the attempts at removal a radial tear in the CCC was noted. All but 1/8th of the segments were removed before the tear extended posteriorly and this remaining fragment was lost.

Action: Ocutome clearance of vitreous and cortex achieved without further untoward events. The section was enlarged to 7.0 mm and a 7.00 mm optic, 13.5 mm diameter IOL was easily implanted in the sulcus; the wound was sutured and a subconjunctival injection of cefuroxime given.

Postoperative medication: Diamox, predforte 1%, chloramphenicol all 4 times daily.

Progress: Day 1: satisfactory, quiet, comfy. Patient informed of problem and complication.
Day 5: 'aching and sore', visual acuity CF, 1.6 mm white hypopyon, no fibrin, cells++, capsular debris, vitritis (see Fig. a).
Treatment: readmitted, given guttae predforte 1% hourly.
Day 6: minimal discomfort; organizing hypopyon, wound oedema, IOP = 20 mmHg
Day 7: settling, vitreoretinal opinion sought. Advice 'watch and see!'.
Day 8: comfortable, VA = 6/60 (see Fig. b).
Day 11: VA = 6/24.
Day 12: VA = 6/18, VR opinion 'leave to resolve'.
Day 15: VA =6/18, fragments resolving.
Day 30: VA = 6/6. Quiet, off all treatment (see Fig. c).

Comment: Rapid onset of severe inflammation following loss of lens fragment into the vitreous cavity settled with topical steroids and acetazolamide. The early interest of the vitreoretinal team was obtained remembering that larger fragments may require surgical removal to prevent glaucoma and cystoid macular oedema.

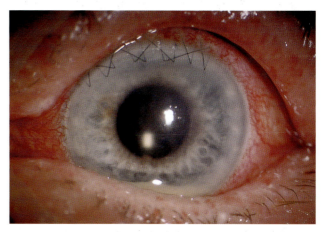

Fig. (a) Inflammation and photophobia, with a small hypopyon

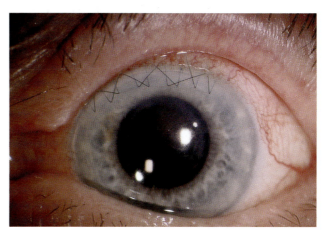

Fig. (b) Resolution of inflammation has begun

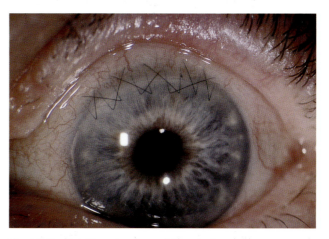

Fig. (c) Comfortable and seeing well 6 weeks later

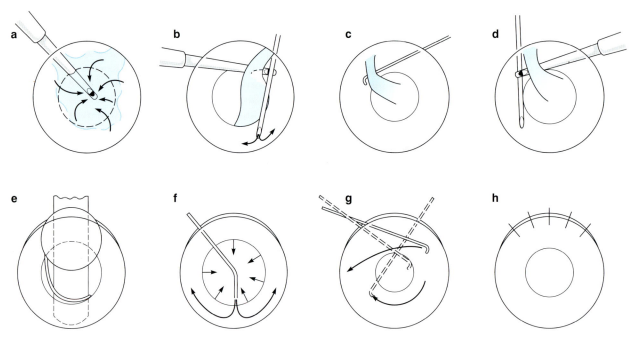

Fig. 4.29 Technique of anterior vitrectomy

5 Introduce the infusion cannula into the second incision (e.g. Butterfly IV cannula) directing the flow away from the rent in the capsule and vitreous (Fig. 4.29b).

6 The anterior CCC should be left untouched. It will provide a shelf for an IOL to sit on.

7 The vitrectomy should continue until the anterior segment is clear of vitreous.

8 Towards the end of the procedure, the infusion cannula can be used to sweep the port of the vitrector to ensure that there is no strand uncut in the hand-piece (Fig. 4.29c). Strands of vitreous, like spaghetti, are cut better at right angles as opposed to in their axis. Clear both inner openings by changing the entry port of the vitrector (Fig. 4.29d).

9 After vitrectomy, the incision is opened to implant an IOL (Fig. 4.29e) (see Chapter 5). The wound should be checked for vitreous strands. If present, further vitrector use anterior to the IOL may be required.

10 Acetylcholine (Miochol) is used to constrict the pupil (Fig. 4.29f). If the pupil is peaked or resists constriction, a careful search will often reveal strands closely applied to the iris surface or lipping up to the wound (Fig. 4.29g).

Once the surgeon is content that the wound is clear, the section should be closed with the preferred suturing technique for ECCE (Fig. 4.29h). A swab can be dragged along the closed wound to look for deformation of the pupil and identify previously silent strands of vitreous. If small, these

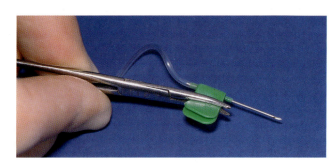

Fig. 4.30 The tabs of a butterfly IV cannula are folded back and held in a pair of artery forceps

can dealt with by gentle traction and excision. Significant wicks will require further anterior segment vitrectomy.

Aspiration phase

Once the majority of nuclear material has been removed complications tend to become easier to manage and have better outcomes. During irrigation/aspiration it is very easy to snag the capsule in the aspiration port. A sudden shearing movement once this has happened will either create a hole in the posterior capsule or unzip a length of zonules causing a dehiscence. The management of a posterior capsular hole has been dealt with earlier in this chapter and the techniques of anterior vitrectomy can be applied here.

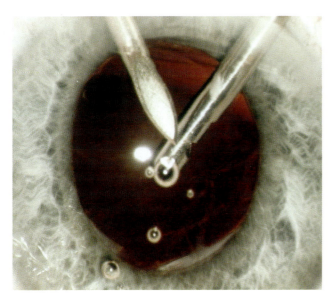

Fig. 4.31 The infusion and vitrector are seen in the eye. Because the infusion is separate, it can be directed away from the capsular hole thus avoiding vitreous hydration and prolapse

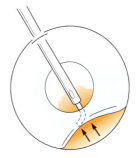

Fig. 4.32 Grade 1 zonular dehiscence

ZONULAR DEHISCENCE (ZD)

In a normal eye, ZD may develop following the use of shearing, tangential forces needed to spin the nucleus without adequate hydrodissection, through the heavy-handed use of the phaco probe without adequate power, or overzealous infusion/aspiration. It is more common with large, hard lenses and in elderly eyes undergoing prolonged surgery.

ZD is usually first noted towards the end of the capsular clearing of cortical lens matter. As the I/A tip is drawn centrally, out of the capsular fornix, a segment of the equator of the capsule will be seen to transiently follow the probe (Fig. 4.32). By releasing the vacuum, the capsule flips back without danger. This can be considered as grade 1 zonular dehiscence and represents around 1 to 2 clock hours of rupture. Provided the surgeon is careful, grade 1 ZD is not a contraindication to implanting an IOL.

If this snagging of the capsular equator is not noticed and the probe is withdrawn before releasing the vacuum the

dehiscence can extend. In grade 2 ZD, the capsule does not 'flip' back when released but remains wrinkled. There is usually greater than 2 clock hours of ZD and consequently the surgeon is better implanting an IOL with loop haptics. These will act as a capsule tension ring. Any foldable lens with loop haptics (e.g. C-loop 13 mm Acrysoft IOL) can be inserted, first into the anterior chamber and then manipulated into the capsular bag using a bimanual technique. This will avoid the shearing forces of dialling.

Grade 3 ZD is where a larger arc of ZD is associated with vitreous prolapse. A vitrectomy will be needed. If there is less than 180° of rupture, it should be possible to stabilize the bag with a capsule tension ring (Fig. 4.33) and to insert any lens with loop haptics such as a one-piece PMMA phaco IOL into the bag.

When performing an anterior vitrectomy with a grade 3 ZD the surgeon should aim to amputate the vitreous at the level of the capsular plane. There is little benefit and much potential danger in attempting to pass the cutter into the posterior segment. It is pointless trying to replace the vitreous using viscoelastics or to repair the dehiscence with a suture.

Grade 4 ZD, which is also associated with vitreous presentation, is where greater than 180° or 6 clock hours of zonule has been ruptured. In EZW cases, where the remaining strands of zonules may themselves be weak, it may be prudent to remove the remaining capsule and opt for a sclerally or iris-sutured lens. If one pole of the capsule is well tethered, it may be possible to place a capsule tension ring into the bag and then to fix the free pole to the sclera with a retaining prolene suture. Once this has been achieved, a one-piece PMMA phaco IOL can be carefully implanted into the bag.

IOL IMPLANTATION

The choice of IOL and the method for its implantation will depend on the surgery that precedes it. This surgery may be routine phacoemulsification, routine ECCE, phaco to ECCE conversion or a complicated case requiring a salvage procedure. The method for converting from phaco to ECCE

Box 4.8 Grades of zonular dehiscence

▶ Grade 1   1–2 clock hours of ZD
▶ Grade 2   2–6 clock hours of ZD without vitreous presentation
▶ Grade 3   2–6 clock hours of ZD with vitreous presentation
▶ Grade 4   Greater than 6 clock hours of ZD

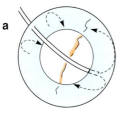

a

After the capsulorhexis, thoroughly hydrodissect the nucleus cortex

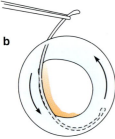

b

The capsule tension ring readily follows the line of the capsule

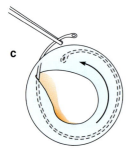

c

Pronate and push backwards. A Sinskey hook may sometimes help positioning the ring

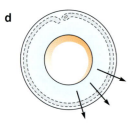

d

The capsule tension ring helps support the dehiscence

Fig. 4.33 Inserting a capsule tension ring using a bimanual technique

surgery will be discussed in the following chapter. Once all potential surgical outcomes have been discussed, the techniques of implantation can be more readily understood (Chapter 7).

Problems with IOL implantation where all preceding surgery has been uncomplicated are principally those of position. The lens may end up in the sulcus instead of the bag. This may not be immediately apparent but the way to check is to snag the anterior CCC with a hook. If this is impossible it is usually because the optic is lying anterior to the capsule. Sulcus fixation with ECCE can alter the refractive outcome but rarely leads to other problems.

This is because of the size of an ECCE lens – 13.5 mm diameter. Phaco lenses are smaller and have not been designed to span the ciliary sulcus. Thus while lens position may appear central while the patient is lying down, it may slip inferiorly when the patient is upright. This may lead to spherical and chromatic aberrations and an unhappy patient.

Provided a round CCC can be seen anterior to the optic, the lens can be assumed to be in the bag. Distortion of the CCC can be caused if one of the haptics is lying in the sulcus. Once the pupil constricts, this will be difficult to notice. As the capsule fibroses with time, contractural forces may lead to decentration of the lens with its attendant refractive consequences.

The lens may be damaged during implantation. Cracks or loss of components away from the visual axis that will not affect the long-term stability of the lens can be ignored. With more serious damage, especially that affecting the visual axis, it is best to exchange IOLs there and then. A lens with an optic and haptics can usually be dialled out of the bag. It can help to inject some viscoelastic behind the optic to help this process. Plate lenses are less easy to manipulate but can usually be encouraged out of the bag with the help of viscoelastic. The wound will require enlarging to remove the IOL which consequently means it will need suturing at the end of the procedure.

SUPRACHOROIDAL HAEMORRHAGE

Suprachoroidal haemorrhage is one of the most feared complications of intraocular surgery (Fig. 4.34). The incidence, signs, management and outcomes are presented in Box 4.9.

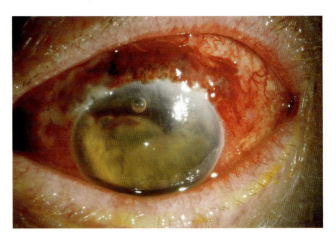

Fig. 4.34 An eye one day postoperatively, following expulsive haemorrhage

Box 4.9 Acute intraoperative suprachoroidal haemorrhage (AISH)

INCIDENCE
- 0.2–0.9% of cataract operations

RISK FACTORS
- Increased axial length
- Raised intraocular pressure

TYPES
- Expulsive
  - spontaneous nucleus expression with extrusion of ocular contents
- Non-expulsive
  - suprachoroidal haemorrhage without loss of ocular contents

SIGNS
- Shallowing of the anterior chamber, loss of the red reflex, extrusion of ocular contents and prolapse of the iris. The majority of AISH occurs after removal of the nucleus

ACTIONS
- Immediate
  - Close the wound quickly and tightly (8/0 or thicker suture material may be required)
  - Perform posterior sclerotomies (1.5 mm in diameter) if the eye cannot be closed
- Later
  - Wait for the clot of any massive haemorrhage to liquefy (which takes 3–5 days) and then drain with posterior sclerotomies under constant infusion pressure

OUTCOMES
- Around 33% will require a secondary surgical procedure
- 20% will attain a postoperative vision of 6/12 or better
- A poor visual outcome of CF or worse is often seen where there has been spontaneous nuclear expression or where vision is only PL at first dressing
- A favourable visual outcome is more common with AISH complicating phacoemulsification as opposed to standard extracapsular surgery (this is probably due to the speed of wound closure with consequent containment of the haemorrhage)

Chapter 5

Converting from phacoemulsification to extracapsular cataract extraction surgery

INTRODUCTION

Cataract surgery can be compared to piloting an aeroplane. The completion of planned, routine surgery is like a perfect landing on the runway. Difficulties encountered during routine phaco surgery may convince the surgeon to convert to ECCE surgery. This is analogous to a safe landing on the grass alongside the runway. However, complications during the operation may be such that a salvage procedure is required – an emergency landing because one of the engines has failed.

Opening the eye to covert from phaco to ECCE is not the same as doing a controlled, planned ECCE. It implies abandonment of the original surgical plan and the need for an escape route to complete the operation. Incisions have to be enlarged, the capsule opened, the lens removed and the wound then has to be sutured. You may have to deal with prolapse of vitreous into the anterior chamber. These added surgical manoeuvres result in an extended postoperative recovery period and the added likelihood of induced astigmatism (Box 5.1).

Because phaco is taught as a closed-eye surgical skill, it is important also to learn the principles of managing the eye if the operation has to be changed into an open eye method because of surgical problems.

WHEN TO CONVERT

The threshold at which an individual surgeon decides to abandon phaco will depend upon his level of competence.

Box 5.1 Problems associated with converting from phaco to ECCE surgery

▶ Creating the ECCE section from phaco wounds
▶ Difficulty in removing the lens
▶ Duration of surgery
▶ Wound closure, suturing, security and stability of wound
▶ Postoperative astigmatism
▶ Poorly compliant patient on the table (movement, coughing)
▶ Slower visual rehabilitation
▶ Expulsive haemorrhage more likely

Control of the CCC may be lost by an inexperienced surgeon but regained by a more experienced one. The more able the surgeon, the higher the threshold which can be considered for conversion.

When a situation is reached where it is unlikely that further progress can be sustained with the phaco approach, it is safer to change to ECCE. This is usually when technical difficulties have occurred in one of the stages or when visualization has deteriorated (Box 5.2).

In the presence of such difficulties, it is better to make the decision to abandon the phaco plan and convert the operation electively. The earlier this decision is taken, the less damage or further problems will accrue.

Box 5.2 Reasons for conversion to ECCE

- ▶ Planned conversion during learning
- ▶ Loss of control or radial tear of CCC
- ▶ Lens too hard
- ▶ Machine failure
- ▶ Loss of confidence/lack of experience
- ▶ Loss of view, poor corneal clarity
- ▶ Pupillary constriction
- ▶ Iris damage
- ▶ Capsular hole with prolapse of vitreous

MODIFYING THE INCISION

There are three wound types usually used to perform phacoemulsification; scleral tunnel, superior clear corneal and temporal clear corneal. All three wounds can be converted to a superior posterior corneal incision for ECCE. This recommended technique is applied to each of the sections that might have been used, with variations that depend on the initial choice.

Cutting an extended corneal wound in an eye which has been previously opened is significantly more difficult. The eye is soft which makes accurate wound construction technically much more demanding. The previous phaco incisions will interfere with the siting and structure of the new incision.

In order to create an acceptable incision certain principles should be obeyed. The eye must be firm before attempting any further manipulation. The new wound must be long enough to allow the nucleus to be expressed and to allow an ECCE-sized IOL to be implanted. The internal opening should consequently have a cord length of at least 10 mm (depending on the size of the nucleus). The incision should be cut in such a way that it aids maintenance of the anterior chamber while completing the surgery and stable when closed with sutures. The safest wound to convert is the phaco tunnel and if you know you are going to convert at the start of the operation, e.g. when teaching, this would be the preferred incision.

GENERAL PRINCIPLES OF WOUND MODIFICATION

The principal steps for constructing the wound are set out below together with special variations for each of the usual phaco incisions.

If the original phaco wounds leak, you should close them with 10/0 nylon.

The anterior chamber is then reformed with viscoelastic and/or BSS (Fig. 5.1a). The eye must be firm.

The projected wound is marked out with the tip of the diamond (Fig. 5.1b). Holding the blade at right-angles to the surface of the eye, a partial thickness stab is made at 2 o'clock. This becomes the fixation point for the forceps (the paracentesis wound can be used for traction if appropriately positioned) (Fig. 5.1c).

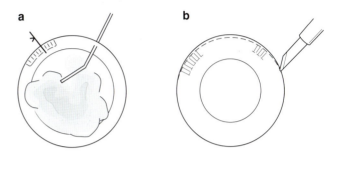

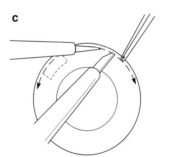

Fig. 5.1 Wound conversion

This incision is then extended at two-thirds depth circumferentially around the superior cornea for approximately 120°, aiming the tip of the knife towards the centre of the eye.

The corneal lip of the wound is opened with forceps allowing visibility of the depth of the initial groove. The wound is now completed by gently running the diamond blade through the base of the wound, aiming at the centre of the pupil.

You should check that the wound is of even depth and of adequate length. The internal opening will have a shorter cord length than the outer. If the initial groove is cut with the blade aimed at the centre of the pupil rather than the centre of the eye, the wound will shelve considerably which will accentuate any internal–external disparity. This problem will be even worse if you simply use a keratome to extend the plane of the original phaco incision (Fig. 5.2).

The wound must be large enough to allow nuclear expression (see Chapter 3). The internal opening should be measured before attempting nuclear expression and

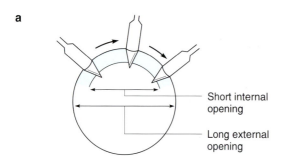

Short internal opening

Long external opening

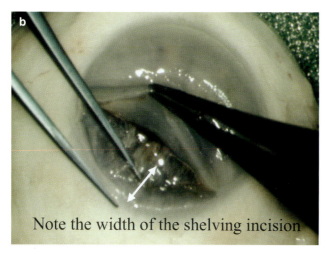

Note the width of the shelving incision

Fig. 5.2 (**a**) Cord length differences between the internal and external openings. (**b**) Long shelving incision created by a misdirected groove (cadaveric eye)

should be a minimum of 10 mm to allow easy passage of all sizes of nucleus (Figs 5.3 and 5.4).

If the wound is too short, it will be impossible to express the nucleus (Fig. 5.5a). Continued pressure in this situation

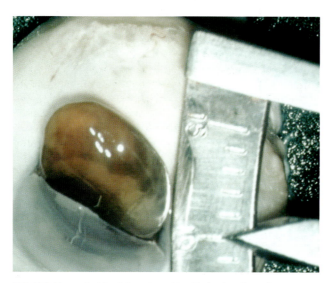

Fig. 5.3 Measuring the internal cord length (cadaveric eye)

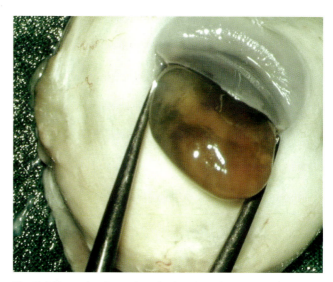

Fig. 5.4 Expressing the nucleus (cadaveric eye)

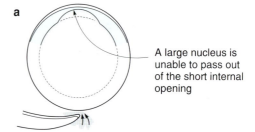

A large nucleus is unable to pass out of the short internal opening

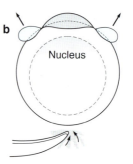

Nucleus

Vitreous prolapses around the nucleus. When the wound is enlarged, the lens within its capsule will be delivered

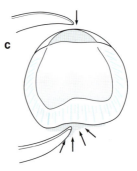

If the wound is too small, the forces exerted during the attempt to express the lens damage the zonule and are transmitted to the vitreous

Fig. 5.5 Problems with expression if the wound is too small

can lead to zonule rupture and vitreous prolapse around the nucleus (Fig. 5.5b, c). Opening the wound after this has happened is like shutting the stable door after the horse has bolted. The opportunity for a complication-free conversion is gone, leaving the surgeon in a difficult position. Expression may be impossible, vectis removal is fraught with problems and an anterior vitrectomy is required.

Phaco tunnel

This wound is the easiest to convert and for this reason it is the authors' incision of choice when teaching. The wound is usually sufficiently watertight and distant from the cornea to allow a corneal section to be cut without problems with the internal openings of the tunnel. The tunnel may need to be closed with a box suture (see Chapter 3) if difficulty is experienced in firming the eye.

Because the phaco wound is not involved in the corneal incision, the section can be cut as if one is performing an ECCE on a virgin eye (see Chapter 3).

Temporal corneal incision

The stab tunnel should be closed with an infinity suture (see Chapter 3). The eye is reformed and the cornea incised superiorly. The wound should be constructed avoiding the original keratome stab.

Superior corneal stab incision

The new incision is started beyond the second or paracentesis incision. It should be extended through the bed of the second incision, around the corneal edge toward the large corneal tunnel. Care should be taken to cut only through the roof of this or a loose tag of cornea will result. The wound can be extended beyond the original corneal stab, further round the circumference, if required.

With either of the corneal phaco incisions, it is tempting merely to widen these, joining the 'phaco' incision to the 'second' incision with the diamond knife or keratome. If performed this way, the resulting incision will be sloping, unstable and difficult to close (see above).

MANAGEMENT OF THE CAPSULE

The CCC, either intact or with radial tear, needs to be enlarged to allow the removal of the lens. Fine Vanna's scissors or Long Ong's scissors should be used to cut two relieving incisions into the capsular opening (Fig. 5.6). If this is not done, then the need to express the nucleus forces may disrupt the capsule or wrench the lens from

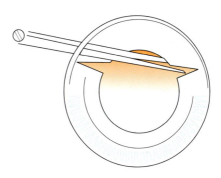

Fig. 5.6 Capsular relieving incisions

its zonule. Gentle hydrodissection should be attempted if vitreous is not presenting.

REMOVAL OF THE NUCLEUS

Assuming satisfactory capsular opening and wound size, expression of the lens should be straightforward.

The eye is grasped at 12 o'clock, 5 mm behind the superior limbus, using toothed forceps. As you push steadily towards the centre of the eye, the superior lip of capsule will be seen to slide back over the superior equator of the lens. Using a second pair of toothed forceps, counter pressure at 6 o'clock, pushing close behind the limbus and directing this force towards the centre of the eye, will prolapse the nucleus (Fig. 5.7). When the lens is through the pupil, you can rotate and brush it out of the eye.

Where there is doubt about the integrity of the zonules, or where a radial tear has extended to the equator, lens expression may result in further problems. The use of an irrigating Vectis forceps will allow a less traumatic delivery of the nucleus into the anterior chamber. From here the lens may be spooned out on the vectis, hooked out with a Sinsky hook or viscoexpressed with viscoelastic (Fig. 5.8). The nucleus can be gently rotated out of the capsular bag using a pair of hooks. Once in the anterior chamber it can be expressed with gentle pressure at 6 o'clock.

The anterior chamber should be immediately reformed with BSS. A careful inspection should be made of the state of the posterior capsule. If intact, the operation can proceed as for a routine ECCE as described in Chapter 3. Capsule deficits will invariably result in prolapse of vitreous into the anterior chamber. An anterior vitrectomy will then be required before assessing the position and amount of remaining capsule which will determine the implantation method and IOL.

ANTERIOR VITRECTOMY

An anterior vitrectomy will be required whenever vitreous presents. The procedure will also allow the safe removal of

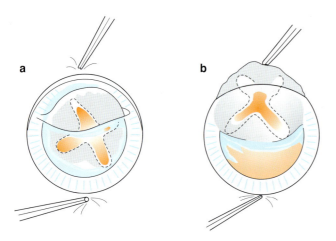

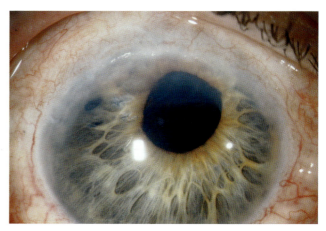

Fig. 5.9 Vitreous incarceration leading to a peaked pupil and anterior uveitis

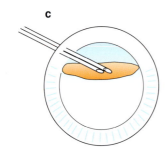

Fig. 5.7 Nuclear expression during conversion

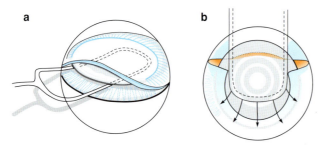

Fig. 5.8 Use of the irrigating vectis

vitreous, lens fragments and cortex and divides connections between the anterior segment structures and the retina. Failure to understand why this is necessary and what happens if not done adequately is to underestimate the long-term pathological consequences of vitreous incarceration, which include cystoid macular oedema, retinal detachment and chronic uveitis (Fig. 5.9).

The technique of anterior vitrectomy is a fundamental skill for any ophthalmic surgeon. If the surgeon feels comfortable with the method and its purpose, then the complication of capsule rupture and vitreous loss will always be competently handled. Familiarity in the use and setting up of vitreous cutting machinery is mandatory.

A vitreous cutter is essential to avoid retinal traction and to complete the toilet of the anterior segment. It is dangerous to merely swab the surgical wound with sponges and cut away the presenting vitreous strands with scissors. The end result of this is to leave vitreous incarcerated in the wound.

Once the IOL has been implanted (see Chapter 6), acetylcholine (Miochol) is recommended to constrict the pupil. If the pupil is peaked or resists constriction, a careful search will often reveal strands closely applied to the iris surface or lipping up to the wound.

Once the surgeon is content that the wound is clear, the section should be closed with the preferred suturing technique for ECCE (see Chapter 3). Dragging a swab along the closed wound and looking for deformation of the pupil can identify previously silent vitreal strands. If small, these can be dealt with by gentle traction and excision. Significant wicks will require further anterior segment vitrectomy.

Box 5.3 Preferred technique for anterior vitrectomy

1 Reinflate the eye using viscoelastic (heavy or normal).

2 Enlarge the second incision by half a diamond-blade's width, angling it to face the inner opening of the principal phaco incision. This will give a wider arc for the vitrector. It will afford an opportunity to remove any last strands of vitreous from the wound at the end of the operation.

3 Pass the vitrector through the rent in the capsule into the anterior vitreous (see Fig. 4.29a).

4 Begin cutting (≥360 cuts per minute) drawing the vitreous in the anterior chamber, posteriorly.

5 Introduce the infusion cannula into the second incision (e.g. Butterfly IV cannula) directing the flow away from the rent in the capsule and vitreous (see Fig. 4.29b).

6 The anterior CCC should be left untouched. It will provide a shelf for an IOL to sit on.

7 The vitrectomy should continue until the anterior segment is clear of vitreous.

8 Towards the end of the procedure, the infusion cannula can be used to sweep the port of the vitrector to ensure that there is no strand uncut in the handpiece (see Fig. 4.29c). Strands of vitreous, like spaghetti, are cut better at right-angles as opposed to in their axis. Clear both inner openings by changing the entry port of the vitrector (see Fig. 4.29d).

9 After vitrectomy, the incision is opened to implant an IOL (see Fig. 4.29e; see also Chapter 6). The wound should be checked for vitreous strands. If present, further vitrector use anterior to the IOL may be required.

10 Acetylcholine (Miochol) is used to constrict the pupil (see Fig. 4.29f). If the pupil is peaked or resists constriction, a careful search will often reveal strands closely applied to the iris surface or lipping up to the wound (see Fig. 4.29g).

▶ Once content that the wound is clear, the section should be closed with the preferred suturing technique for ECCE (see Fig. 4.29h). Drag a swab along the closed wound to look for deformation of the pupil and identify previously silent strands of vitreous. If small, these can be dealt with by gentle traction and excision. Significant wicks will require further anterior segment vitrectomy.

Chapter 6

Lens implantation in difficult circumstances

INTRODUCTION

Once implanted, an IOL should not need either to be adjusted or changed postoperatively. Surgery should not proceed unless the surgeon is happy with the lens style and power for that patient. Fashion, knowledge, technologies and information change constantly and surgeons are under constant commercial pressure to choose or use this lens material or that style. This makes it hard to know which is the best IOL. Whilst there is often little to choose between one lens and another, it is usually best to avoid unusual designs and experimental materials. It should be remembered that the IOL will be in place for many years and it may be better to choose a lens made out of a material with a lengthy track record.

The use of foldable lenses is now well established. Although there is less long-term follow-up of acrylic lenses, their superior biocompatibility with respect to silicone IOLs and the reported lower incidence of posterior capsular fibrosis may make them the foldable lens of choice. IOLs will vary not only in material but also design. The optic and haptics may be fashioned from the same piece of material (one-piece lens), or be combined with prolene haptics or PMMA haptics (three-piece lens).

PMMA remains the material of choice for rigid phaco or ECCE lenses. The surface of these lenses can be modified with adsorbed heparin that inhibits inflammatory cellular deposits. These are particularly useful in eyes that have suffered from uveitis and may suffer further inflammation postoperatively. Following capsular rupture or conversion from phaco to ECCE, the size and style of IOL is important. If the haptic to haptic diameter is too small (e.g. phaco IOL measures 10.5 mm overall), the lens will wobble in the ciliary sulcus, the so-called windscreen-wiper effect. A lens that has long flexible haptics has better circumferential contact with the sulcus and consequently gives better support. This is crucial where parts of the capsule or zonule are missing (Box 6.1).

IOL implantation must be slick, and the insertion uncontaminated. In the routine case, lens insertion is just another

Box 6.1 Potential difficulties with IOL implantation

▶ Difficult insertion
▶ Lens damage
▶ Wrong lens power
▶ Loss of normal support, e.g. posterior capsule
▶ Capsule/zonule damage by the IOL
▶ Lens implantation after converting

part of the operation, but, when things have gone awry, knowing how and what to do is important to ensure satisfactory pseudophakia. The problems of lens insertion, position and damage are discussed in turn.

DIFFICULTIES INSERTING IOL

Many problems of insertion are caused by trying to force the lens through too small an incision. Each lens has a finite size and this will determine the minimum size of incision required for insertion. Foldable IOLs of higher dioptric powers need a larger incision. Even though the diameter of the optic may measure 6 mm, the incision must be large enough to accommodate their bulk, and must be larger than half of the optic diameter. Whether flat or folded the incision must be big enough to easily admit the IOL.

Attempting to squeeze the IOL through a tiny wound will either be impossible or cause damage to the wound architecture, making it more likely that the wound will leak. The resulting precipitate delivery of the IOL into the eye is extremely dangerous as the lens can be driven through the posterior capsule. Counter-traction on the lip of the wound by forceps can tear these thin tissues, and at the end of surgery the wound will not be watertight and will require suturing. Better to slightly overestimate wound length in the first place rather than finding out that this will have to be done later when the lens is held folded in forceps in the dominant hand. If the wound does need to be enlarged, it is important to inflate the eye with BSS or cutting will be difficult or lack precision.

LENS DAMAGE DURING INSERTION

It may be stating the obvious to say that before implantation every lens must be checked for blemishes and structural faults, but the removal of a damaged lens, particularly a folding lens, is not straightforward. Whereas the section will have to have been large enough to permit implantation (or explantation) of a rigid lens, the incision for a folding lens is typically much smaller than the diameter of the IOL inserted. Consequently, in order to remove a folding lens, the wound has either to be adequately opened or the lens cut up inside the eye and removed piece-meal. Cutting the lens is difficult because the IOL slips easily out of the jaws of the scissors. By enlarging the incision to approximately 5.5 mm, the lens can normally be easily dragged out of the eye and replaced with another lens of same or quite different design.

The wound will probably need to be sutured.

Fracture of the lens, especially the softer silicone plate-haptic lenses, is not an infrequent problem. If the crack does not extend across onto the optic of the lens and there is sufficient haptic remaining to ensure stable fixation, the lens may be left in the eye. If the visual axis is affected or if the stability is threatened, the IOL should be removed.

PROBLEMS OF POSITIONING THE IOL

Sometimes the haptics of the IOL fail to enter the capsule as intended. This happens more often when the pupil is small, and it is not easy to see where the IOL is going. If implanted into the sulcus it is possible that the lens will sag away from the visual axis – the so-called setting sun sign. When implanted with only one haptic in the sac, the lens optic will be displaced by the forces of contraction driven by the anterior capsule joining to the posterior (when both legs are lying in the bag, the forces are concentrically resisted and the lens will stay put).

Using a bimanual technique it is usually possible to get the whole IOL into the bag. The loop haptics are compressed by two hooks, e.g. Kuglan and Sinskey, and then by gentle rotation of the lens and posteriorly directed pressure both the legs and then the optic can be guided into the sac (Fig. 6.1).

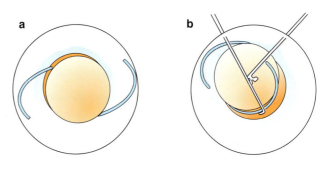

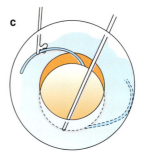

Fig. 6.1 A bimanual technique is used to ensure in the bag implantation of the IOL. (**a**) The haptics have missed the CCC and are lying in front of the capsule. (**b**) Push backwards on the optic with a Kuglan hook, and use a Sinskey hook to flex the haptic and gently introduce it into the bag. (**c**) Rotate the IOL pushing it lower in the bag. Engage the upper loop with the Kuglan hook and compress this haptic. As the lens is gently dialled, the haptic will pop into the sac

LENS IMPLANTATION AFTER CONVERTING WITHOUT VITREOUS LOSS

After converting from phacoemulsification to ECCE, the skills needed for IOL implantation are similar to those following routine ECCE surgery; the IOL to be used will be the same as used for ECCE. Any tear in the capsule will be exaggerated by the expression of the nucleus. In phaco surgery, the higher pressures can lead to posterior extensions of these tears; this is seen less often during complications of ECCE surgery.

1 Check the wound has been enlarged sufficiently to let the lens pass through it.

2 Inflate the lower fornix of the capsule with viscoelastic.

3 Holding the IOL push the leading haptic into the bag.

4 Take the upper loop near its tip and whilst gently rotating the whole lens clockwise, pronate the hand. This will bend the upper haptic and slide this into the upper sulcus of the capsule. (The pronating procedure has exposed some difficulties for left-handed surgeons.)

5 Alternatively, with a Kuglan hook, flex the upper haptic downwards towards the optic of the lens;

then push the point of the Kuglan backwards and at the same time twist the hook. This will free the haptic which will now flick up into the upper sulcus or capsule.

Ensure that the IOL is stable, that the optic is lying centrally and that the legs are not wrapped in vitreous.

Refer back to Figs 3.21 to 3.24 for basic technique.

LENS IMPLANTATION AFTER COMPLICATED SURGERY

After complicated cataract surgery the problem of implantation has to be considered. A range of options is available with the choice being determined by the remaining structures available for supporting the lens. The IOL may be fixed in the capsular bag or left in the ciliary sulcus; where there is insufficient capsular support, the lens may be placed in the anterior chamber or sutured posteriorly to the iris or sclera. In some circumstances, the IOL may already be in the eye when a complication develops.

Decide how the lens is to be supported in the eye, i.e. sulcus, capsule, anterior chamber (see Table 6.1). Choose a lens of the correct power and size. If you decide to place the lens in the sulcus it must be at least 13 mm in length.

IOL implantation, where there is insufficient capsule for sulcus fixation, requires experience. If there is any doubt as to whether there is sufficient capsule for stable sulcus support, or where an implanted lens appears unstable, it is better to remove the IOL, close the eye and plan for implantation as a secondary procedure.

Capsular bag

This is always the preferred option if there is sufficient capsule. Whilst relatively easy to insert the IOL into the bag after either routine phaco or ECCE, after a stormy surgical passage the capsular bag is usually damaged making

it difficult to place the IOL within it. Occasionally it is possible to implant a lens in the bag with a complete posterior/anterior tear but this is achieved with difficulty and danger (Fig. 6.2). Simpler methods are available.

A simple radial tear should not prevent in-the-bag implantation (Fig. 6.3), but it may be best to avoid unfolding the lens within the capsule as any rip may extend. The IOL can be unfolded in the anterior chamber and then gently dialled into place. Align the haptics so that their spring is directed away from the tear (Fig. 6.4). Plate IOLs are contraindicated because of the risk of posterior dislocation through an unseen hole in the capsule.

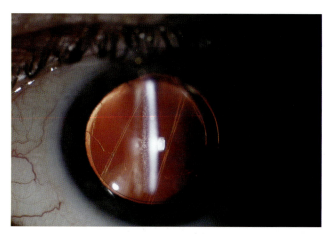

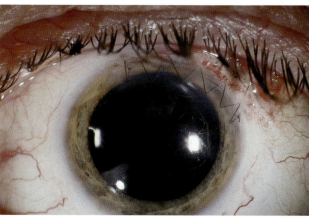

Fig. 6.2 The IOL lies comfortably within the capsule, but a complete tear of both anterior and posterior capsule is noted

Table 6.1 Options for IOL implantation

Procedure/complication	Implantation option
Routine phacoemulsification	Implantation into bag
Routine ECCE	Implantation of IOL in bag/sulcus
Routine conversion to ECCE	Implantation of IOL in bag/sulcus
Small hole in posterior capsule	Sulcus fixated IOL with optic in bag
Large hole in posterior capsule	Sulcus fixation of 13.5 mm IOL
Large radial tear	Sulcus fixation with lens axis at 90° from the tear
Large capsular tear, remaining rim	Sulcus fixation with Sheet's glide
More than 50% of capsule lost	Anterior chamber
	Sutured (iris, sclera)
	Contact lens

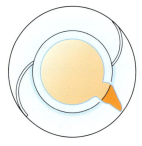

Fig. 6.3 A simple radial tear should not prevent in-the-bag implantation

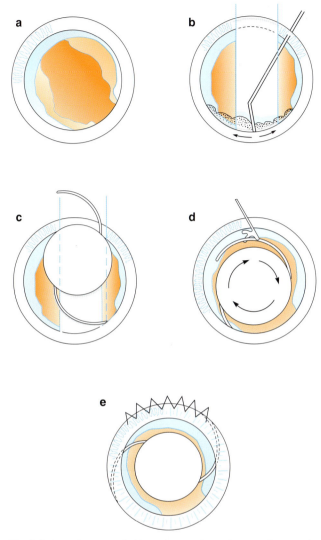

Fig. 6.4 A tear has extended from the anterior to the posterior capsule. The IOL can be guided into the sac with a Sheet's glide and dialled into a position away from the tear

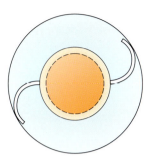

Fig. 6.5 A folding lens of 13 mm will usually lie safely in the sulcus

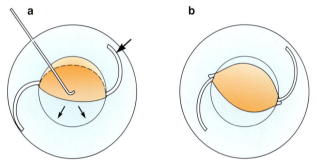

Fig. 6.6 The 'buttonhole' method to stabilize a sulcus-fixated lens

Sulcus fixation or combined CCC/ ciliary sulcus fixation (buttonhole method)

After total disintegration of the posterior capsule, the anterior capsule and the CCC may remain. The lens can then be safely implanted into the ciliary sulcus (Fig. 6.5). If the eye is big (for example, highly myopic) or if the IOL is shorter than the diameter of the sulcus, there is a risk that the lens will lie low in the pupil.

Combined CCC/sulcus fixation: to centrally fix an IOL with loop haptics, the optic can be popped through the CCC, leaving the haptics in front of the capsule and the optic behind (Fig. 6.6). To achieve this most elegantly, the CCC needs to be slightly smaller than the lens optic.

The CCC will end up lozenge shaped, with a good capsular opening. If the aperture in the CCC is too small after the optic has been buttonholed, a 'cat's eye' effect will result, which is not acceptable. Try enlarging this with a combination of scissors and tearing – not an easy task.

This 'buttonhole' method is also useful if, after introduction of a folding IOL into the sac, the posterior capsule is found to be damaged and unsuitable to support the IOL. In this situation the legs will now be posterior to the CCC and the optic is now fished forwards through the CCC, trapping it there (Fig. 6.7). If the CCC is too small, it is not possible to enlarge it, then the whole lens will have to be brought forwards into the precapsular space or ciliary sulcus. Neither method is appropriate for use with plate-haptic lenses.

The capsule can still be used as support provided there is more than 200° of circumferential rim remaining. This may be difficult to estimate at the time, and if in doubt, the

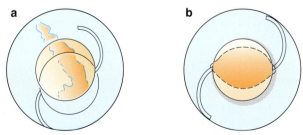

Fig. 6.7 The posterior capsule has disintegrated as the IOL is inserted. The lens is dropping into the posterior segment. By bringing the optic forward through the CCC, the lens is stabilized

eye can be closed and implantation performed as a secondary procedure a week or two later. By this time, the capsular remnants will be more easily visible and stronger because fibrosis will have started to form.

The ideal IOL for sulcus fixation should be at least 13 mm long to span the eye and have C-shaped haptics to afford maximum contact with the remaining capsular shelf and sulcus.

Implanting the IOL into the ciliary sulcus

1   Open the section to accommodate the lens of choice.

2   If required, complete the anterior vitrectomy and check there is no vitreous to the wound.

3   Inject viscoelastic under the corneal dome and into the superior and inferior fornices.

4   Place a Sheet's glide into the inferior sulcus.

5   Introduce the IOL along the top of the glide and position the upper haptic with a Kuglan hook.

6   If the capsular remnants are sparse, use a Kuglan hook instead of dialling or pronating.

7   Complete the operation by suturing etc.

Insufficient capsule for sulcus fixation: anterior chamber lens implantation

Anterior chamber implantation is the least technically demanding procedure but needs to be done well to avoid the many problems for which the technique is infamous. It is most important to use a lens of the correct size. The difficulty is that when the eye has had an anterior vitrectomy it is partially collapsed and attempts at measuring the horizontal diameter of the cornea will underestimate the real size needed.

To avoid these problems, remember to make the measurements *prior* to carrying out the vitrectomy (a counsel of perfection) or fully inflate the eye with BSS before using the calipers. Check the white to white horizontal corneal diameter and add 1 mm to get the size of anterior chamber lens.

Anterior chamber IOLs should probably be reserved for older patients, where the duration of endothelial attrition will be less. It is best performed as a secondary procedure because measuring the open eye for an ACIOL tends to inaccuracy. Lenses that are too big will press into the vital structures in the angle, causing chronic uveitis with accompanying pain and tenderness (Figs 6.8 and 6.9). Vision may be compromised in the long term by cystoid macular oedema.

When the ACIOL is too small (Fig. 6.10), the lens will rotate about its longitudinal axis, damaging the angle struc-

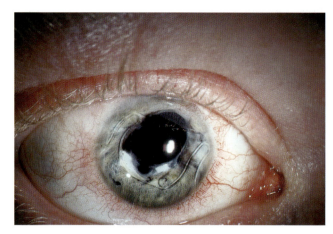

Fig. 6.8 An intensely inflamed eye following implantation with an anterior chamber IOL that is too long

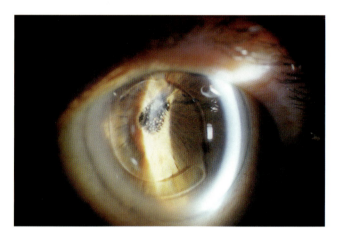

Fig. 6.9 This oversized IOL is bowed backwards and covered in inflammatory cells

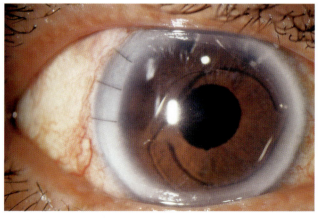

Fig. 6.10 When the anterior chamber IOL is too small, the lens will move around in the anterior chamber. Note that this lens is lying freely in the anterior chamber

tures, and rattle against the endothelium of the cornea leading to cell loss and eventual bullous decompensation.

The possible complications of angle damage and endothelial loss makes the choice of an ACIOL a higher risk option unless the cardinal points of their use are respected.

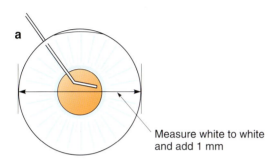

Measure white to white and add 1 mm

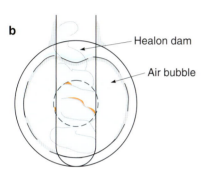

Healon dam

Air bubble

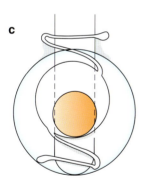

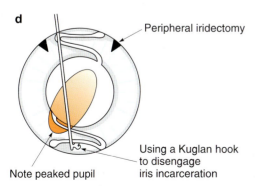

Peripheral iridectomy

Note peaked pupil

Using a Kuglan hook to disengage iris incarceration

Fig. 6.11 Implanting an anterior chamber IOL

THE TECHNIQUE OF ANTERIOR CHAMBER IMPLANTATION (Figs 6.11, 6.12)

1   Measure the horizontal diameter of the cornea (white-to-white distance) and add 1 mm. This gives the physical size of the implant that will best fit the eye (range 11.5–13.5 mm). Use a Kelman-style 'multiflex' lens.

2   Fill the anterior chamber with air.

3   Check for vitreous strands up to the wound by sweeping with a fine cannula. Any movement or distortion of the pupil whilst doing this indicates that vitreous remains.

4   Perform a further anterior vitrectomy if vitreous remains in the anterior chamber.

5   Inflate the anterior chamber with viscoelastic.

6   Pass a Sheet's lens glide into the opposite angle.

7   Place viscoelastic on the anterior surface of the lens glide to help the lens through the surgical wound.

8   Insert the IOL, but aiming the legs of the lens slightly anteriorly so that iris root is kept clear of the haptic.

9   Withdraw the lens glide.

10 Compress the proximal loop with a Kuglan hook, inserting the elbow and then the tip of the haptic over the lip of the corneal wound.

11 Observe whether the pupil is round or ovalled; the pupil should be round and move independently when the sclera is probed. If the pupil is peaked towards one of the haptic points, the iris will have to be freed from around it.

12 Free the iris by compressing the leg of the lens and lifting it slightly forwards. This should encourage the incarcerated iris to slip out, and the pupil will quickly return to its round shape. (If the lens is too long, the pupil will remain oval even after the tips of the lens have been disengaged from the iris in the angle. It must be exchanged for a lens one size

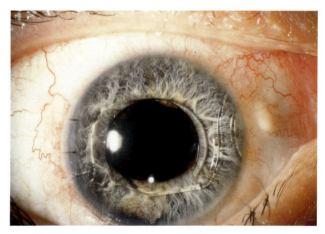

Fig. 6.12 An optimally situated anterior IOL

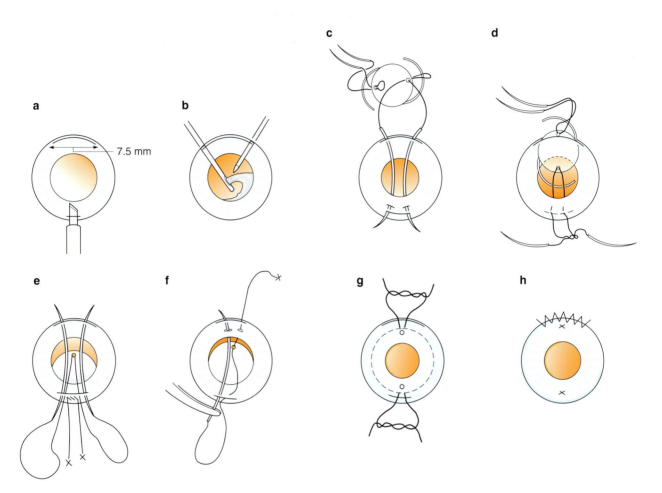

Fig. 6.13 Iris-sutured PC IOL: long needles on 10/0 prolene are tied through the dialling holes on the optic and are passed across the anterior chamber, through the mid-periphery of the iris and tied. The process is repeated with another pair of needles, but this time the needles are first passed back to front and then back through the superior, mid-periphery of the iris. The knots are tightened and completed when the IOL is snuggly positioned behind the iris

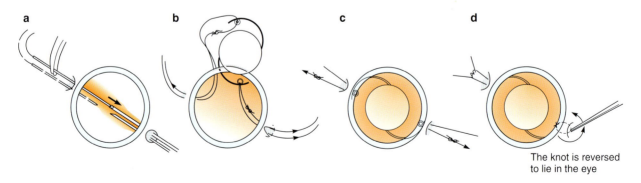

The knot is reversed to lie in the eye

Fig. 6.14 Sclerally sutured PC IOL: long needles on 10/0 prolene are tied to the haptics of the IOL and passed behind the iris to pierce the sclera either through the ciliary sulcus or through the pars plana, immediately behind the ciliary body. The thread is tied and the knots buried or rotated so that they lie either in the eye or under scleral flaps

smaller. If it is too small, the lens will be unstable and will slip from the position it has been placed in.)

13 Inject Miochol to constrict the pupil and to check that the lens and iris are free one of the other.

14 Perform a peripheral iridectomy to avoid pupil block glaucoma.

15 Remove any viscoelastic.

16 Record the postoperative axis of the lens such that, at a later date in the clinic, any lens movement can be appreciated and documented.

17 Close the corneal wound with a continuous 10/0 nylon suture.

Posterior chamber implantation in the absence of sufficient capsule requires that the lens is either sutured to the iris or the sclera. In a situation where a surgeon loses posterior capsule and vitreous and finds himself wanting to implant a backup lens, if an anterior chamber lens is not available or there is insufficient capsule support, suturing the lens to the iris is possible even with such a soft eye. These techniques are part of the repertoire of advanced anterior segment reconstructive surgery and should only be performed by an experienced surgeon or by a senior trainee under supervision by the same. The techniques are shown in outline in Figs 6.13 and 6.14.

There is much to be lost and little to be gained by attempting implantation when in surgical difficulties. It is better to wait, explain the problem to patient and/or consultant and reassess the eye for implantation as a secondary surgery, a few weeks later.

Chapter 7

Postoperative problems and their management

INTRODUCTION

The patterns of postoperative review will vary as much as the surgical techniques themselves. Some surgeons review their patients the day after surgery and then at 1 week. Some prefer telephone contact the following day and clinical review at 2–3 weeks. An individual's practice will depend on unit policy and the confidence he or she has in their surgery.

The recovery from routine cataract surgery is usually straightforward. Whilst the patient's eye might be red and feel gritty, the improvement in vision outweighs these complaints and the patient is generally happy.

The examination routine for postoperative visits should be focused to look for any potential complications. The eye is usually tender to touch and photophobic hence an extended, comprehensive examination is uncomfortable. The clinician should concentrate on obtaining an accurate visual acuity, with and without a pin-hole. The wound is examined for leaks, the cornea for oedema, the anterior chamber for cells or flare and the pupil for regularity. The intraocular pressure should be checked and a quick retinal examination performed with a 90D lens. The pupils should be dilated and examined more fully if there have been surgical problems. Poor vision can indicate problems with IOP, retina or the IOL which should be checked for position and stability.

Problems may present later on the day of surgery or at a later date in the convalescent period.

Complaints later on the day of surgery are principally of pain. This may be due to corneal abrasion which may follow a slow recovery in lid function after anaesthesia. A deeper ache may indicate anterior chamber collapse or suprachoroidal haemorrhage. Ocular paraesthesia as the anaesthetic wears off may cause distress unless the patient is warned beforehand.

A bloody serous 'leak', noticeable on the pad or running down the cheek, may too cause considerable anxiety and often only requires simple reassurance.

Certain problems and complications will become obvious at different times during postoperative recovery (see Box 7.1; Table 7.1). Complicated surgery is often followed by a less predictable convalescence and for this reason these patients should be reviewed by the surgeon at regular intervals.

The day after surgery patients may complain of poor vision, diplopia or pain. Persistent mydriasis may be the only cause for reduced vision. In this case the patient can be reassured that acuity will improve over the following couple of days. A displaced or subluxated IOL, or one of the wrong power, should allow respectable pin-hole

---

Box 7.1 Problems presenting later on the day of surgery

▶ Corneal abrasion
▶ Raised intraocular pressure (IOP)
▶ Leaking wound
▶ Suprachoroidal haemorrhage

Table 7.1 Postoperative examination

Structure	Finding
Lids	Abnormal function
Ocular movements	Mechanical restriction/palsy
Conjunctiva	Haemorrhage
Wound	Phaco burn, leak
Cornea	Oedema, Descemet's folds, abrasion
Anterior chamber	Inflammation, vitreous, lens matter
Iris	Irregular pupil
IOP	Hypotony, hypertension
IOL	Position, stability
Retina	Check if no view preoperatively

vision. If the patient is essentially aphakic in the visual axis, the use of a +12 dioptre lens with the pin-hole will allow a more accurate vision to be recorded.

Corneal oedema, retained lens matter and vitreo-retinal pathology will lead to reduced vision which cannot be corrected with a pin-hole. Preoperative strabismus, with or without diplopia, can lead to binocular double vision after surgery. Muscle damage at the time of local anaesthesia may have the same result. Monocular diplopia can be caused by a subluxed IOL, folds in the posterior capsule or by macular pathology.

Corneal epithelial damage leads to sharp pain, for example, corneal abrasion or epithelial bullae. Most gritty-type pain is epithelial in nature and will settle rapidly. Diabetics tend to have more persistent problems with epithelial healing defects. The pain of uveitis is a deeper ache that will not be relieved by a drop of local anaesthetic. A significant pressure rise characteristically leads to a bony pain in the eyebrow.

Much of the pathology discovered the day after surgery (see Box 7.2) may continue to cause problems for the days and weeks to come. Some postoperative complications develop later and these include endophthalmitis, cystoid macular oedema and lens deposits (see Boxes 7.3 and 7.4).

Box 7.2 Problems presenting the day after surgery

- Diplopia
- Corneal oedema – localized or generalized
- Raised IOP
- IOL wrong power/position (aniseikonia)
- Wound leak
- Iris prolapse
- Vitreous prolapse
- Uveitis/iritis
- Retained lens matter – cortex or nuclear
- Vitreous haemorrhage – anaesthetic perforation
- Hypopyon/endophthalmitis
- Suprachoroidal haemorrhage

Box 7.3 Problems presenting within the first week (see also Box 7.2)

- Uveitis
- Endophthalmitis
- Glaucoma
- Corneal oedema

Box 7.4 Problems presenting 1–8 weeks after surgery

- Persistent uveitis
- Cystoid macular oedema
- Lens deposits
- Raised IOP (secondary to steroid or inflammation)
- Persistent corneal oedema
- IOL power and refractive surprises
- Astigmatism
- Capsular phimosis
- Retinal problems, e.g. detachment, macular disciform
- Posterior capsular fibrosis

CORNEAL ABRASION

Peribulbar local anaesthesia may cause a prolonged period of lid paralysis and poor lid closure. Corneal and conjunctival desiccation follows and commonly causes an oval epithelial defect in the inferior half of the cornea. A single eye pad may aggravate the problem as the eye will open under the dressing. Care should be taken when padding the eye after surgery to ensure that the lid is closed. The use of a plastic shield which is completely covered in tape will allow humidity to rise which can prevent corneal drying and help patient comfort.

TREATMENT

The patient should be encouraged to close the eye if possible. Local anaesthetic and antibiotic ointment such as chloramphenicol can be used if the eye will not close easily or the patient is uncomfortable. The patient should be reassured that the problem is only minor and will resolve rapidly.

RAISED INTRAOCULAR PRESSURE (IOP)

A transient pressure rise probably occurs in many patients without either symptoms or signs. This is usually self-limiting but may persist for a day or two after surgery. If the pressure builds slowly it causes little or no symptoms. The surgeon should expect raised IOP when surgery has been difficult or where there is a history of glaucoma (Box 7.5). These cases should be treated prophylactically

Box 7.5 Causes of raised IOP in the immediate postoperative period

▶ Retained viscoelastic
▶ Dislocated lens fragment
▶ Pre-existing glaucoma
▶ Secluded/occluded pupil with iris bombé
▶ Uveitis
▶ Hyphaema
▶ Expulsive haemorrhage

with intravenous or oral acetazolamide which can be tapered postoperatively.

If symptomatic, raised IOP may lead to reduced vision due to corneal oedema or a pain which is often described as a bony ache in the eyebrow. Retained nuclear fragments can lead to high postoperative pressures and a brisk inflammatory response.

TREATMENT

Whatever the cause, symptomatic ocular hypertension in the immediate postoperative period requires medical treatment. So too does an IOP of 30 mmHg or above with or without corneal oedema. Unless there has been a stormy surgical course, problems with IOP are usually short-lived and respond to a short course of topical beta-blockers or a few tablets of oral acetazolamide (standard- or sustained-release).

Pressures above 45 mmHg are very rare in the absence of retained nuclear fragments. Temporizing measures to reduce IOP should be attempted whilst waiting for surgical removal of retained material. Oral or intravenous acetazolamide should be given immediately and 6-hourly after this. If the IOP does not settle in the first 1–2 hours, an osmotic agent should be tried (e.g. mannitol 1–2 g/kg body weight of a 20% solution) or if the first-line treatment is poorly tolerated or ineffective. Nausea, caused by the glaucoma, can be alleviated with oral or parenteral prochlorperazine (Stemetil) and pain may be eased by sublingual or parenteral opiates.

Unexplained or persistent IOP problems may be the result of steroid response. Steroids should be stopped and the patient reviewed a week or two later. Where there is a history of glaucoma or ocular hypertension, a non-steroidal anti-inflammatory preparation should be used postoperatively.

POSTOPERATIVE HAEMORRHAGE

Blood in the anterior chamber

Transient perioperative haemorrhage regularly occurs when cataract surgery has been combined with a drainage procedure. It also occurs in cases of Fuch's iridocyclitis as the anterior chamber is entered at the beginning of the operation (Amsler's sign). Most anterior chamber haemorrhage will clear within a day or two and will only cause problems if it becomes trapped behind the IOL.

Bright red blood in the vitreous

Globe perforation from the needle of the local anaesthetic block can lead to vitreous haemorrhage. The blood is usually bright red and vision reduced to CF or worse. There may be a history of pain during the administration of the local anaesthetic or of topping up of block. A B-scan ultrasound examination should be performed.

TREATMENT

Early referral to a vitreo-retinal surgeon should permit the recognition and treatment of a major problem. Delay can be dangerous and may lead to retinal fibrosis. Sub-retinal blood is a poor prognostic feature for visual outcome.

Dark red blood or loss of the red reflex

This is a bad sign and strongly suggests that there has been an ophthalmic disaster, i.e. a suprachoroidal haemorrhage (Fig. 7.1). The patient will usually have experienced pain

Worked Example 7.1

A highly myopic 58-year-old woman.

Peribulbar anaesthesia failed to produce akinesia and hence she had a further injection in the upper nasal quadrant. Postoperatively, she was NPL with a bright red reflex. There was no RAPD but a retinal detachment was possible on the B-scan. She was referred to a vitreo-retinal surgeon.

She underwent a pars plana vitrectomy with drainage of the SRF. Sub-macular haemorrhage was noted but no puncture was found. Her final VA was 6/24 best.

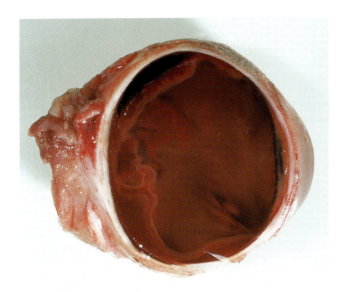

Fig. 7.1 Enucleated eye showing suprachoroidal and vitreous haemorrhage following ocular perforation

and may be seeing at best light perception or hand movements. The anterior chamber will be shallow and there may be prolapse of iris or more tissue. A dense afferent pupillary defect will be seen. B-scan ultrasonography will confirm the findings (see also Box 7.6).

LEAKING WOUND

With small incision surgery, a leaking wound and a shallow anterior chamber should not occur. Slow leaks with a formed anterior chamber can simply be observed but may occasionally require a bandage contact lens.

Large wounds, wounds that are poorly constructed or those that have suffered surgical trauma (e.g. phaco burn) may leak briskly and lead to loss of the anterior chamber. This should be obvious at the first postoperative examination. The patient's eye will usually be injected, the vision poor and choroidal effusions may be seen. If there has been loss of all aqueous for some hours, the ciliary body may be in shock, which may cause an artificially negative Seidel dye test.

TREATMENT

If the anterior chamber needs reforming the patient should be taken back to the operating theatre and the wound sutured aseptically. This is also the case where a leak is brisk even if the anterior chamber is formed. A bandage contact lens may be applied whilst arranging an appropriate theatre slot. Injecting BSS or air at the slit-lamp is uncontrolled and dangerous and does not address the problem of the leaking wound.

CORNEAL OEDEMA

The use of viscoelastics during phaco surgery protects the endothelium from the damage of ultrasonic energy and high flow rates. Despite this precaution, corneal oedema can still occur (Box 7.7). This oedema can complicate routine surgery when there is pre-existing endothelial pathology. It can also result from poor surgical technique when the cornea was originally healthy.

It may be localized to the wounds or to an area overlying the main activity of the phaco tip or it may be generalized and diffuse. Descemet's membrane stripping will cause a localized patch of oedema above the defect but can lead to a more diffuse effect as hydrostatic pressure forces fluid between the stromal lamellae.

TREATMENT

Raised IOP may contribute to postoperative corneal oedema and should therefore be treated. Absolute or relative endothelial failure, with or without folds in Descemet's membrane, can often resolve with conservative management over a couple of weeks.

If the phaco probe or second instrument has stripped Descemet's membrane, efforts should be made to replace it with the injection of a bubble of SF_6 gas (see Chapter 5). Repair of Descemet's membrane is shown in Figure 7.2.

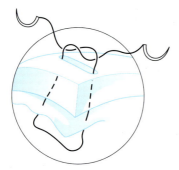

Fig. 7.2 Repair of Descemet's stripping by through and through suturing with double ended 10/0 prolene. The knot is buried in a partial thickness corneal slit

Oedema and Descemet's folds that persist for more than 6 weeks rarely clear spontaneously. Whilst the use of hypertonic (5%) saline drops or ointment can sometimes alleviate both symptoms and signs, these eyes often require a corneal graft to restore vision.

IOL PROBLEMS

Problems with the implant are a major reason for secondary surgical interventions and medicolegal challenges. Complications must be detected early and an explanation and plan of action discussed with the patient. Problems fall into two categories: the wrong power and the wrong position.

Wrong power

The first clue is poor vision on the first postoperative day. If acuity improves with a pin-hole, a refraction will confirm the error. A shallow anterior chamber with an anterior shift of the lens/iris diaphragm may lead to an apparent myopic surprise. At the 1- or 2-week review, the exact extent of the discrepancy can be formally assessed and a decision made whether to persevere or proceed with a lens exchange.

Inaccurate biometry may lead to an inappropriately powered implant being used. The result may be intolerable anisometropia. Whilst there may be some refractive drift, differences of greater than 3 dioptres between eyes are usually symptomatic.

TREATMENT

In the short term, occluding one lens of the patient's spectacles may help. Definitive treatment for intolerable anisekonia will be IOL exchange, supplementary intraocular or contact lenses or refractive surgery. IOL exchange should be undertaken within 3 or 4 weeks (Figs 7.3 and 7.4). After this time, the capsular bag becomes fibrosed, making intracapsular exchange impossible.

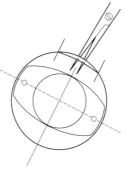
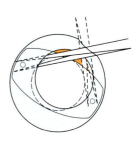

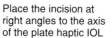
Place the incision at right angles to the axis of the plate haptic IOL

Use Long Ong's scissors to divide capsular adhesions through the positioning holes on the IOL

Fig. 7.3 Removing a plate lens: adhesions between anterior capsule and posterior capsule through the dialling holes will need to be divided with long fine scissors

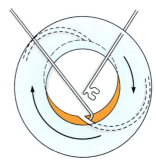

Fig. 7.4 Removing a three-piece IOL by dialling with a Sinskey hook. A second hook can be used to apply counter pressure to the capsule to prevent it from disinserting from the zonule

Malposition

Small displacements of the IOL were frequently seen after ECCE where the haptic's final position, either in the bag or in the sulcus, was uncertain. IOL malposition is less common following uncomplicated phaco surgery. Where there has been iris damage or an incomplete CCC, tissue entrapment by a misplaced IOL is more likely. Malposition is due to poor placement at the time of surgery and not movement overnight! Involvement of the iris will cause a deformed pupil and often a low-grade anterior uveitis.

The IOL may be poorly centred inside the capsular bag which may indicate retained viscoelastic. These situations will often self-correct.

Damage to the posterior capsule during surgery may have left an incomplete platform for the IOL but the use of a large optic implant with long flexible haptics will give better stability (see Chapter 6). If it is inadequate, the lens may partially or totally dislocate. Partial dislocation will result in a decentred lens which will cause refractive problems including prismatic and spherical aberration (Fig. 7.5).

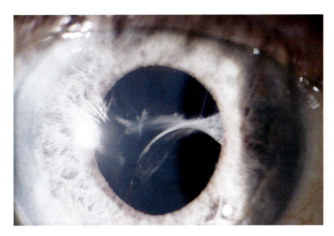

Fig. 7.5 Setting-sun sign. In this case the IOL has slipped through a deficient zonule

If the IOL dislocates totally, it will come to lie in the vitreous or on the inferior retina. The patient will then be rendered effectively aphakic.

TREATMENT

A malpositioned lens is commonly poorly tolerated by the patient. If the patient is symptomatic or if you are concerned that the position of the IOL will cause problems, lens exchange should be considered. The risks of any secondary procedure to secure the IOL in its proper place must be weighed against any potential damage the surgery might cause. If there is iris entrapment, the IOL should be repositioned as soon as possible to avoid pain, uveitis and cystoid macular oedema.

The second procedure required depends on the amount of remaining posterior capsule. If there is greater than 180° of capsular rim, an unsutured sulcus-fixated IOL can be used. Without this support, alternative fixation is required, i.e. anterior chamber IOL or a sclerally or iris-sutured posterior chamber lens. A completely dislocated IOL sitting on the retina can be left and the patient re-implanted depending on the remaining posterior capsule. Alternatively, it may be removed by floating it up on heavy liquid as part of a pars plana vitrectomy procedure.

At the time of surgery, or in the day or two following it, it can be difficult to quantify the remaining capsular support. Within a couple of weeks the residual capsule will opacify making it much easier to assess. Providing you are sufficiently confident, re-implantation can be planned.

UVEITIS

Mild anterior chamber inflammation is seen in the first 24 hours after the majority of cataract surgery. Where surgery has been prolonged or traumatic, the proteinaceous component of any inflammation may increase. If severe, this may form fibrils of fibrin which may coalesce in the pupil. Visual acuity will fall and will be impossible to improve with a pin-hole.

Retained lens fragments should be suspected whenever an inflammatory response is brisk or persistent.

TREATMENT

The routine use of topical steroids or non-steroidal anti-inflammatory drugs is usually sufficient. The anti-inflammatory effect may be heightened by changing the preparation (e.g. betamethasone to dexamethasone) or increasing the frequency or concentration. Sub-conjunctival and sub-Tenon's injections are rarely needed.

Fibrin can get enmeshed with retained viscoelastic, resulting in a particularly sticky combination that can take weeks to clear completely. Inflammation that increases during the postoperative period or appears at day 3 may indicate the development of endophthalmitis.

ENDOPHTHALMITIS

Whilst uncommon following routine cataract surgery, endophthalmitis can be a devastating complication that may blind the eye. The most common time for presentation is 5–10 days postoperatively, although the definition of acute endophthalmitis is of a panuveitis within 6 weeks of surgery. The incidence, organisms, presentation, diagnosis and management of endophthalmitis is presented in Tables 7.2 and 7.3.

The diagnosis of chronic endophthalmitis is often delayed because the uveitis is steroid-responsive. If the inflammation returns on reducing topical treatment, you should have a low threshold for suspecting chronic infection and a vitreous tap is mandatory.

VITREOUS PROLAPSE

Vitreous will tend to move from high to low pressure. Strands and knuckles will be drawn towards the wound. Vitreous may traverse the wound – a vitreous wick – or become incarcerated in it. Wicks are often associated with aqueous leaks leading to hypotony. Pupils may be irregular due to sphincter rupture or phaco damage but vitreous incarceration should be excluded by careful examination.

There should be no vitreous in the anterior chamber following uncomplicated cataract surgery. Occasionally, vitreous strands may pass between the zonules in a highly myopic eye. The most common cause for vitreous in the anterior chamber is incomplete vitrectomy at the time of complicated primary surgery. The pupil will be peaked where a strand of vitreous has passed around the edge of the iris up to one of the incisions (Fig. 7.6).

Table 7.2 Endophthalmitis

	Post-traumatic	Acute postop	Chronic postop
Incidence	Overall 7% Rural up to 30%	Cataract 0.07–0.13% Drainage 0.06–1.8%	Not available
Organisms	*Staph. epidermidis* *Bacillus cereus* *Streptococcus* spp.	*Staph. epidermidis* (70%) *Staph. aureus* (10%) *Streptococcus* spp. (9%) Gram-negative organisms (6%)	*Staph. epidermidis* *P. acnes* *Candida* spp.
Presentation	Pain, photophobia Intense pain Panuveitis Hypopyon Afferent pupil defect Poor vision	Pain, photophobia Discharge, reduced VA Chemosis, injection Anterior and posterior uveitis and hypopyon Afferent pupil defect Within 6/52 of surgery	Persistent low-grade uveitis Post-capsular plaque – *P. acnes* More than 6/52 post-surgery
Risk factors	Lens disruption IOFB Plant-related injury Delayed primary repair and wound leak	Pre-existing external eye infection, prolonged surgery, vitreous loss/incarceration Wound leak	No specific risk factors known
Diagnosis	Anterior chamber tap and vitreous biopsy	Anterior chamber tap and vitreous biopsy	Excision-biopsy of the plaque

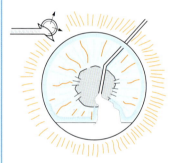 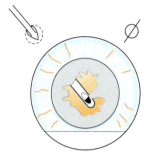 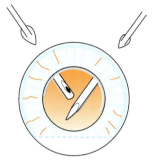 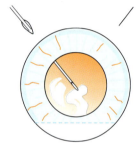

Fig. (a) Aspirate as much fibrinous material as possible using a 27G needle on a tuberculin syringe. The contents are sent for culture. Re-inflate the anterior chamber with viscoelastic attempting to drive open the pupil. Create two scleral flaps 3.5 mm behind the limbus using a circular blade. The eye is opened using a myringotomy blade aiming at the centre of the globe

Fig. (b) Immediately behind the lens/capsule perform an anterior core vitrectomy with a vitreous cutter. Aspirate the macerated vitreous manually through the vitrector using a three-way tap. The contents are sent for culture and microscopy

Fig. (c) If there is a considerable quantity of vitreous debris, a more extensive core vitrectomy can be performed using a butterfly cannula for irrigation

Fig. (d) Antibiotic is injected (see drugs and dosages below). The bevel of the needle faces upwards and the injection is carried out slowly. The wounds are not sutured

	Post-traumatic	Acute postop	Chronic postop
Treatment	Amikacin Vancomycin (synergistic for *B. cereus*) Oral prednisolone for all cases if inflammation is severe	Ceftazidime Vancomycin Dexamethasone (intravitreal and sub-conjuctival)	Vancomycin Amphotericin B (for fungi)
Outcome	Poorest outcomes 30% better than 20/400	Depends on organism: 20/100 or better with *S. epidermidis* 84% Gram negative 56% *Staph. aureus* 50% Streptococci 30%	Good visual prognosis
Prophylaxis	Prompt primary repair Early use of antibiotics (as above) Removal of all foreign material	Preop. topical quinolone antibiotics 5% povidine-iodine preparation	As for acute endophthalmitis

P. acnes = Proprionibacterium acnes.

Table 7.3 Recommended treatment dosages for endophthalmitis

Early vitrectomy may improve the visual prognosis. Antibiotics are best made up with 0.9% NaCl solution, except amphotericin when 5% dextrose should be used

Intravitreal	Ceftazidime	1.0 mg in 0.1 ml
	Vancomycin	1.0 mg in 0.1 ml
	Amikacin	0.4 mg in 0.1 ml
	Amphotericin	5.0 mcg in 0.1 ml
Topical	Cefuroxime 5% forte, half-hourly, alternating with gentamicin 1.5% forte for the first 24 hours, then reduce (use gentamicin if fulminating infection and pseudomonas suspected) Alternatively, Ofloxacin/Ciprofloxacin	
	Econazole	if fungi suspected
Oral	Ciprofloxacin	750 mg b.d.
	Fluconazole	200–400 mg b.d. if fungi suspected
Intravenous	Amoxycillin/Flucloxacillin	250–500 mg, 6 hourly if necessary
	Amphotericin B	if fungi suspected

Notes: Systemic antibiosis are not required for cases of chronic postoperative endophthalmitis. If the inflammatory response is very brisk use Prednisolone orally (1 mg/kg body weight) for 5 to 10 days.

Reference

Kresloff, M.S., Castellarin. A. A. and Zarbin, M. A. Endopthalmitis: *Survey of Ophthalmology*, **43**(3), (Nov–Dec1998) 193–224. (319 refs).

Worked Example 7.2

A 67-year-old male underwent uncomplicated cataract surgery using an ECCE technique. There was initially an excellent recovery of vision but at 6 weeks, a moderate uveitis persisted. The steroids were increased in strength and frequency with moderate resolution of signs. However, as the drops were tapered off, the inflammation recurred and the patient complained of reducing vision and discomfort. The patient was referred for a second opinion.

At presentation, the visual acuity was 6/60 and the eye was inflamed. Slit-lamp examination showed marked anterior chamber activity, microscopic hypopyon and poor red reflex (Fig. a). After dilating the pupil, a large intracapsular white mass was noted behind the IOL. A provisional diagnosis of chronic endophthalmitis secondary to either *Staphylococcus epidermidis* or *Proprionibacterium acnes* was made.

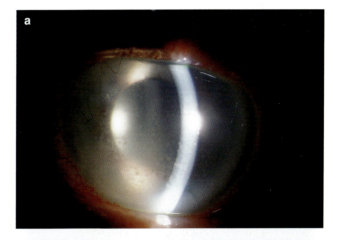

The capsule, IOL and abscess were removed *in toto* through a corneal incision after injection of alpha chymotrypsin (Fig. b). A vitreous biopsy grew *P. acnes*. Intracameral injection of amikacin and vancomycin was given and the patient was treated with intensive topical antibiotics for 6 weeks (see protocol in Table 7.3).

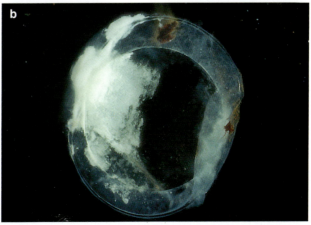

Vision improved to 6/9 (with a +12 lens and pin-hole) following this procedure. A secondary iris-sutured IOL was implanted, resulting in a spectacle-corrected vision of 6/6.

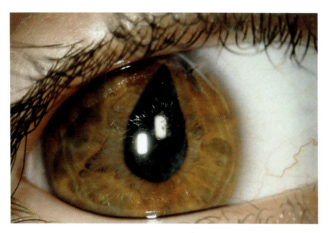

Fig. 7.6 Peaked pupil due to vitreous prolapse

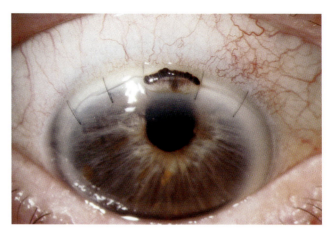

Fig. 7.7 Iris prolapse

If there is a significant 'knuckle' of vitreous in the anterior chamber and the pupil is distorted, this will lead to anteroposterior vitreous traction, retinal hole formation and cystoid macular oedema.

TREATMENT

Vitreous herniating through the wound can create a portal for infection and internal traction forces which can lead to retinal detachment. It does not spontaneously resolve and requires surgical management. The patient should be taken back to the operating theatre where the anterior chamber and wound can be cleared using a vitrector and a bimanual technique.

A small vitreous 'knuckle' floating free in the anterior chamber can be ignored unless it is interfering with the pupil margin.

These eyes, even if managed well, will retain a higher risk of developing a retinal detachment at a later date. The patient should be advised of the warning symptoms for retinal detachment (drop in visual acuity, large or multiple floaters and a sudden onset of a field defect).

IRIS PROLAPSE

Iris tissue, especially if atonic, will herniate through a wound. Iris prolapse is more common with extracapsular surgery where the wound, and potential pressure gradient, is larger. Small herniations may be difficult to see but should be suspected with a peak of the pupil. Incarcerated iris tissue causes pupillary distortion and secondary iritis. This tissue is a potential route for infection and may increase the risks of sympathetic ophthalmia (Fig. 7.7).

TREATMENT

When a limbal/scleral section has been used, the iris herniation may be contained within the wound itself. If it

---

Box 7.8 Causes of iris prolapse

▶ Poorly constructed wound
▶ Poorly repaired wound
▶ Sudden rise in IOP, i.e. trauma or expulsive haemorrhage
▶ Atonic/damaged iris tissue

---

passes through the wound, it will retain a conjunctival cover or become coated in epithelial cells. Provided there is no strangulation, and consequent ischaemia, iris tissue may remain viable indefinitely in this situation.

Ideally, an iris prolapse should be replaced as soon as possible, within one or two days of being discovered. Topical or sub-Tenon's anaesthesia should be used where possible to reduce the risk of increasing IOP with a periocular injection.

Sutures in or around the prolapse area should be removed as they will have been worked loose. Uncovered herniated iris will lose its viability within 24–36 hours, hence after this time it should be excised rather than replaced. If a paracentesis does not already exist, one should be made with a diamond blade. This will allow the iris to be swept away from the wound using a Rycroft cannula (Fig. 7.8). It is sometimes necessary to make a small peripheral iridotomy to decompress an aqueous balloon. The wound should then be resutured with interrupted 10/0 nylon. Topical steroids and antibiotics should be given postoperatively.

RETAINED LENS MATTER

The spectrum of retained lens matter runs from a wisp of soft cortical material to an entire crystalline lens. Whilst it

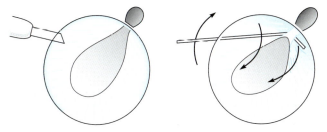

Fig. 7.8 Diagrams showing how to repair an iris prolapse

is one of the major complications of cataract surgery, the management decision tree has few branches. Soft cortical matter and small nuclear fragments (less than a quarter of the nucleus) will usually disappear from the anterior chamber without further complication. Retained material within the capsular bag can however lead to a fibrinous inflammatory reaction (Fig. 7.9). Fragments retained posteriorly often cause more problems with inflammation and secondary glaucoma.

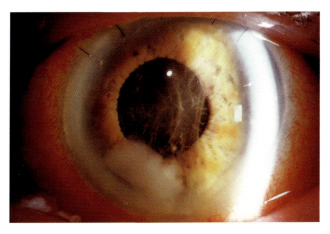

Fig. 7.9 Fibrinous uveitis caused by retained soft lens matter

TREATMENT

Patients must be carefully observed. Small amounts of soft lens matter and nucleus will spontaneously disappear. Provided that the associated uveitis is mild and that there is no secondary glaucoma, surgical intervention is not indicated.

Where there is a brisk uveitis or raised IOP or where a nuclear fragment has fallen posteriorly, the patient should be taken back to theatre. The early support of a vitreo-retinal colleague should be invited so that appropriate surgery can be planned. A second procedure will usually involve a pars plana vitrectomy and floating the dropped fragment up into the anterior chamber with heavy liquid (see Chapter 4).

CYSTOID MACULAR OEDEMA

Cystoid macular oedema (CMO) complicates approximately 3% of routine cataract operations. It is more common where there is pre-existing inflammation, where the fellow eye suffered CMO following surgery or where there is a predisposition to this pathology, for example retinitis pigmentosa. As a late postoperative problem, chronic cystoid macular oedema will be seen in patients with a history of previous complicated surgery involving vitreous loss, iris incarceration and chronic inflammation.

It is the cause of disappointment and anger in patients and frustration in surgeons! It causes a reduction in central vision, which may develop 2–10 days postoperatively. There may be some image distortion and patients characteristically complain of things appearing to look 'red'. The earliest sign is a loss of foveolar detail compared with the fellow eye. Established and usually untreatable oedema collects in bullae giving a petalloid appearance to the centre of the macula. The condition can be elegantly demonstrated by fluorescein angiography and scanning laser ophthalmoscopy (Fig. 7.10).

TREATMENT

The cause for CMO is unknown but is probably inflammatory in nature. The routine use of postoperative steroids can reduce the later incidence of CMO. Topical non-steroidal anti-inflammatory drops (Ketorolac) have been shown to be of benefit in treatment when used four times a day for 90 days. Sub-Tenon's or orbital floor injections of a long-acting steroid (depomedrone) may encourage resolution, which may then lead to less scarring. Oral NSAIDs, such as Froben, may have a role to play and oral diuretics, such as acetazolamide, may reduce the oedematous component.

Patients with retinitis pigmentosa are predisposed to suffer from CMO. This complication often worsens following surgery for one of the other recognized ocular associations – posterior sub-capsular cataract. Routine postoperative treatment should include an orbital floor injection of depomedrone and a 3-month course of oral acetazolamide (125 mg b.d.).

POSTERIOR CAPSULE OPACIFICATION AND FIBROSIS

Thickening and fibrosis of the posterior capsule may be apparent very soon after surgery. It complicates approximately 100% of children's cataract surgery, 50% of young adults' and around 10–20% of operations in the elderly. Opacification risks are reduced for the newer IOL designs and for the newer materials, particularly acrylic composites. Patients complain of decreasing vision, glare or monocular diplopia around 1–6 months after primary sur-

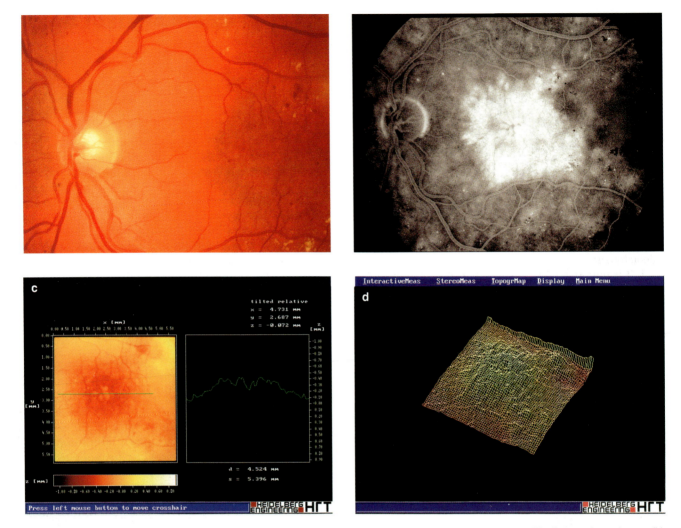

Fig. 7.10 Cystoid macular oedema (**a**) occurring postoperatively in a diabetic patient following complicated surgery. The fluorescein angiogram (**b**) shows classical petalloid oedema which is confirmed on the scanning laser ophthalmoscope photographs (**c**). Note the disturbance in the retinal surface demonstrated in the grid projection (**d**)

Box 7.9 Technique for Yag capsulotomy

▶ Obtain informed consent – there will probably be an increase in the number and size of floaters, the IOL may be damaged, the IOL may become unstable and there is a small, increased risk of retinal detachment

▶ Partially dilate the eye with 0.5% tropicamide (wide dilatation may make it difficult to create a central hole)

▶ Set the laser on defocus (which focuses the laser a fraction behind the aiming beams)

▶ Set the power on 0.5 mJ and fire a peripheral test shot, increasing or decreasing the power according to the reaction

▶ Cut a superior 180° arc around the circumference of the desired-size hole

▶ Complete with an inferior 180° arc

▶ If the total dose is over 50 mJ there is a risk of laser-induced anterior uveitis and it is prudent to prescribe topical low-strength steroid drops for 3–4 days

gery. Problems would be anticipated if a stubborn posterior capsular plaque had been found at surgery.

Posterior capsules are usually symmetrical, with an increased chance of laser treatment being necessary if the fellow eye required it.

TREATMENT

The use of the Nd-Yag laser to perform a posterior capsulotomy is the preferred treatment (Box 7.9). With all lens materials, there is a risk of causing damage (pitting) with the laser. Although opacification rates are lower with acrylic lenses, it is very difficult to create a central gap as the posterior capsule becomes very adherent to the IOL. Laser treatment should be delayed for at least 3 months, and preferably 6, to reduce the risk of inducing a retinal detachment.

If it is impossible to make an adequate opening with the laser, a formal surgical membranectomy will need to be considered (Fig. 7.11a,b).

CAPSULAR PHIMOSIS

The fibrotic process which commonly affects the posterior capsule can extend to affect the whole capsular bag. The associated contracture and shortening associated

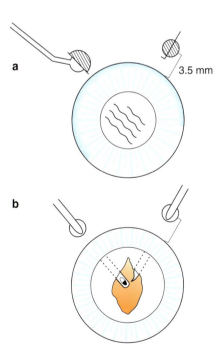

Fig. 7.11 Technique for surgical membranectomy. Two partial thickness scleral flaps are made with a circular blade, 3.5 mm behind the limbus. Insert a myringotomy blade through each of the incisions using one stab to incise the posterior capsule. The vitrector is then used to clear an opening in the capsule. A separate butterfly cannula infusion needle with its tip gently hooked helps to strip an opening in this fibrous tissue

with this process may decentre the IOL or narrow the anterior capsular aperture. If this smaller capsular 'pupil' is drawn eccentrically by continued fibrosis, vision will be compromised.

TREATMENT

Capsular phimosis is better prevented than cured. Tearing a larger CCC will reduce the risks and reduce its clinical effect. Once present, the aim of treatment is to relieve tensions and clear the visual axis. This is best done with the Nd-Yag laser with the defocus switched off (Fig. 7.12a,b). If unsuccessful, formal surgical membranectomy will need to be considered.

LENS DEPOSITS

Anterior IOL inflammatory IOL deposits ('lens measles') are aggregates of macrophages and giant cells that collect on the implant's anterior surface (Fig. 7.13a, b). If observed over time with sequential photography, they can be seen to

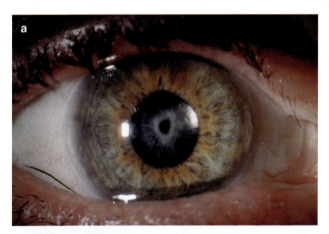

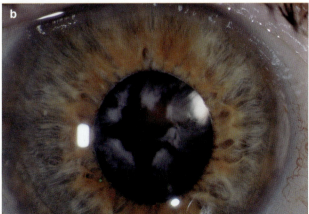

Fig. 7.12 Capsular phimosis in a patient with a plate haptic lens is treated with Yag laser. Four radial slits are cut with the laser with satisfactory reopening of the capsular orifice

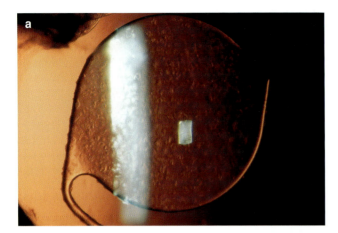

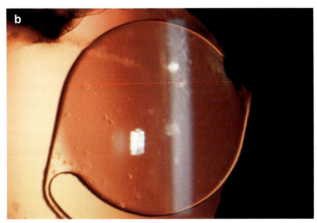

Fig. 7.13 Cellular deposits on an anterior chamber lens (**a**) treated with topical steroids for a month, showing a dramatic improvement (**b**)

move and change position. They are more common where there has been iris damage (including an iridectomy as part of a trabeculectomy procedure).

TREATMENT

The deposits can be removed (polished) off the IOL using the Nd-Yag laser. The laser is set on minimum power (0.5 mJ) without defocus. The aiming beams are focused just anterior to the deposit which is seen to disappear on firing. The deposits will simply reform if the eye is not subsequently treated with topical steroids (guttae beta-methasone four times a day). Drops may need to be continued for weeks or months.

ASTIGMATISM

Small incision surgery has been developed to reduce induced astigmatism and speed up the visual convalescence following cataract surgery.

ECCE needs a long wound, which consequently requires suturing. Sutures that are too loose, or break, will result in wound collapse. This will induce an against-the-rule astigmatism in the axis of greatest sag. Corneal sutures should be left in place for 12 weeks before elective removal to prevent a secondary wound collapse.

Sutures that are too tight will lead to wound compression or over-running. The astigmatism this causes is with-the-rule. Release of the sutures will allow the wound to relax. Removing all sutures before 12 weeks runs the risk of causing a secondary collapse (Fig. 7.14).

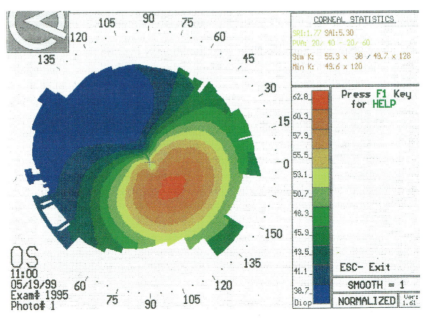

Fig. 7.14 Corneal topographic map showing a high postoperative against-the-rule astigmatism in a patient in whom corneal sutures were needed to close an enlarged wound. Early suture removal at 4 weeks resulted in collapse of the section and a dramatic change in astigmatism

In sutureless phaco surgery, the longer the wound the greater the induced against-the-rule astigmatism. Wounds up to 3.5 mm result in around 2 dioptres of cylinder. Wounds that are longer than this should be sutured to prevent early collapse. Sutures can be removed from short wounds in 3–4 weeks without causing sagging. If the wound has to be enlarged and sutured, it is sensible to wait for 12 weeks before removing the sutures.

TREATMENT

Persistent with-the-rule (WTR) astigmatism can be treated by concentric keratotomies in the axis of the positive cylinder.

Whilst against-the-rule (ATR) cylinders can be treated in the same way, in most cases the wound should be resutured and the use of compression sutures considered (Fig. 7.15).

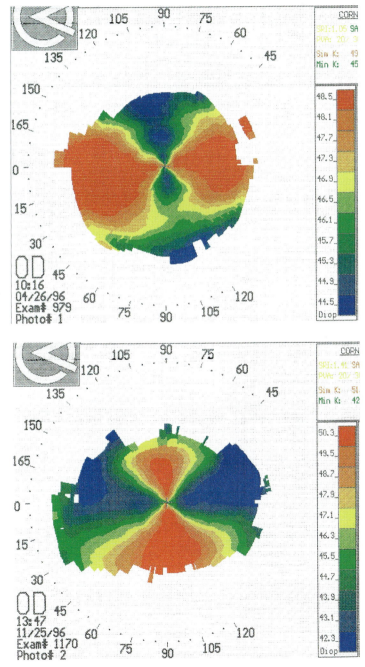

Fig. 7.15 Corneal topography of a patient who had postoperative collapse of her wound after suture infection had caused dramatic against-the-rule astigmatism. The wound was reconstructed by refashioning and resuturing causing a temporary WTR astigmatism which settled when the sutures were removed at 4 months

Part Three

The Doctor–Patient Relationship and Medicolegal Matters

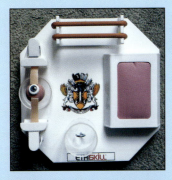

8 Surgical competence and clinical governance

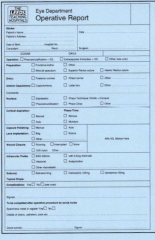

9 Medicolegal matters

Chapter 8

Surgical competence and clinical governance

INTRODUCTION

A physician can no longer survive on clinical ability alone. Even if this were the case, in the practice of medicine today, the words 'clinical ability' would need qualification. The ability of one surgeon to manage a patient's problems may not be matched by another's. The surgeon must understand his or her limitations and be realistic in both what can be expected of their performance in any given case and in what they advise the patient when discussing likely outcomes. The application of the combination of medical knowledge and surgical skill with insight into one's ability, can be thought of as clinical competence.

Remaining within one's own zone of competence is the safest and only justifiable approach. Where a problem requires treatment that is beyond the skills of one ophthalmologist, that patient should be referred to another with special experience or greater ability. In this way the patient is offered the best quality of care, and the greatest likelihood of a successful outcome. In cataract surgery, this suggestion may seem rather overstated, but when reviewing cases for surgery it is clear that some are going to be more difficult than others. It may be more appropriate that the consultant does a particular case or that the advice of a colleague is sought to discuss possible problems that might need specialist intervention in the months postoperatively. They should not be treated merely as a 'routine' case. Certainly, in a firm where there are surgical trainees, the more complex cases need to be separated from the standard risk case and appropriate supervision given.

UNDERSTANDING COMPETENCE

Only appropriately trained or supervised personnel should undertake surgery. Whereas it is easy to measure a doctor's experience, for instance by looking at a training logbook, their actual ability to operate may be limited. For them to understand and express these limits requires insight and honesty. Their competence is measured then by a combination of skill, judgement and integrity. Good surgeons know when and when not to operate or offer treatment. They will know their limits and the limits of the treatment on offer.

Senior surgeons should be able to cope with all the potential complications of the surgery being performed and will be able to use any instrument or machinery necessary for managing a complication. Even difficult or risky cases should be within their grasp. Their skill and experience allows them to be confident in the teaching and performance of their surgery. In a conceptual model they will be unaware of the level of their special skills, and this unconscious competence represents mastery (see Fig. 8.1). On the other hand, when learning to operate (surgical trainee) or learning a new technique (established specialist), all trainees should be aware of their surgical limitations. This awareness of their limitations represents insight, and such conscious incompetence is the entry point to the learning cycle. With the will to learn, this surgeon strives to learn the new technique. There will be mistakes along the way, but with time and application, the technique will be perfected (conscious competence). In time this skill becomes unconscious and at this stage the surgeon has attained mastery (unconscious competence).

Change, for whatever reason, will threaten this mastery. It might be that a new technique comes along, e.g. phacoemulsification, and the experts must accept that they now lack this new skill and must be willing to learn the new method. The learning cycle has shifted and they are no longer the 'masters'. This is a healthy and constructive situation and a state of mind that will serve one well through a long surgical career. If, on the other hand, the driver for change is a loss of skill – perhaps brought about through ill health – the steps to keep up may be too difficult and other solutions will need to be explored.

At the heart of the learning cycle is the understanding of one's limitations and a life-long appetite to keep up to

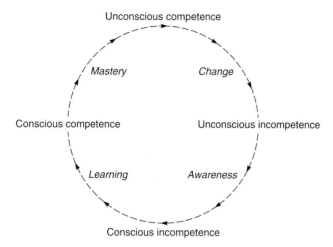

Fig. 8.1 The learning cycle (after JWR Peyton, *Teaching and Learning*, Rickmansworth, Manticore Europe, 1998)

date. Knowing when better methods are around the corner is an invitation to seek opportunities for further training; it is not a reason to pretend that the moderate technique that you practise is adequate or cannot be improved. If insight can be defined as a consciousness of one's situation, a lack of insight in a surgeon is dangerous. Unconscious incompetence leaves the surgeon blissfully unaware of the damage he or she might be about to cause (or have caused). It leaves them without the drivers for improvement. Experience in itself is not sufficient to generate competence. There has to be a commitment to participate in teaching and training.

Any adverse event is an opportunity to the trainer to discuss and explain to the trainee not only the management of the complication but also the need for surgical humility. Stressing the necessity to admit when things have gone wrong may seem painful at first (and it will always be so) but will enable the junior to better cope when problems occur in the future. Video-taping your operations allow you to self-analyse your technique. It will also afford the chance to discuss with a colleague, senior or junior, the way through the problem so that it won't happen again.

No one ophthalmologist can offer a uniformly high level of care in all speciality fields. You will find different grades of competence in the many different aspects of your professional life. Interestingly, a patient's perception of how good a doctor is may be greatly enhanced if, recognizing your own limitations, you refer the patient for a second opinion when you are stuck with a problem of management. It is accepted practice now to refer retinal patients to retinal specialists. In cataract surgery some may feel that cataracts and all the problems and complications that may ensue, lie within the domain of every ophthalmologist, and that therefore it is not necessary to ask for help or even to think that a better way forward can be offered by another. If appropriate, share your problems and grow in the admiration of your patient.

SKILLS ACQUISITION

As surgical practice has drifted from generalist to specialist practitioners, so too has the chance diminished for surgical trainees to obtain the wide surgical training previously available. The skills of cutting a corneal section or handling and tying fine suture materials, for example, are in danger of being lost, as they are not routinely used in phacoemulsification. In consequence, when a junior surgeon is faced with a complication during a cataract operation, an obvious difficulty arises. How can the complication be handled competently when basic skills are either missing or unpractised and knowledge of alternative techniques is not available?

One way forward is to encourage the participation in micro-skills workshops. By identifying and teaching the generic skills in appropriately equipped and staffed 'wet-labs' these deficiencies may be at least partially redressed. Here the training ophthalmologist can be taught the principles of microsurgery, instrument design, suture handling and wound construction and closure. Such skills must be learned by trainees at the inception of their surgical training. Combining this with structured and regular surgical practice, the trainee will be equipped to develop mature and broad skills. Inherent in this approach is the constant need for consultant or specialist help in implementing structured surgical training and experience into already full schedules of service commitments and training programmes.

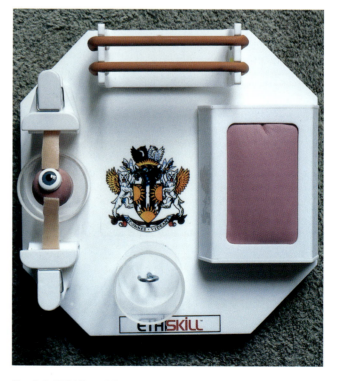

Fig. 8.2 Ethiskills training board

An example of how this can be developed is the initiative taken by the Royal College of Ophthalmologists. It has recognized the high technical entry point to surgery now required of surgical trainees and has established a national basic surgical skills faculty. The faculty will design and deliver courses to doctors in the first year of their training. In conjunction with Ethicon they have designed a 'skills board' (Fig. 8.2) which can be used to encourage the practice of basic surgical skills, either in local wet-lab facilities or when the eye theatre is empty.

CLINICAL GOVERNANCE AND AUDIT

The issues surrounding the supply of quality medical care are becoming increasingly pertinent.

Corporate policies to achieve so-called total quality management were developed in the early 1990s. These policies strove to deliver a customer-focused service revolving around an organization-wide commitment to teamwork and a constant improvement of quality. Quality issues in medicine are more difficult to quantify. Internal measures of success require external comparisons. Benchmarking is the practice of comparing outcome measures between organizations and can generate programmes to find and implement best practice. Benchmarking in the field of health forms the basis of clinical governance.

Research is required to discover what constitutes best clinical practice. Audit can be considered as the investigative process by which we can find out if our clinical practice is in fact the best. Evidence-based medicine is the cornerstone for the production of best-practice protocols.

Clinical governance covers the issues of best clinical practice and risk management. It incorporates approaches to develop guidelines for evidence-based clinical practice and the mechanisms by which these can be disseminated throughout the staff population. With the implementation of continuous professional development and audit feedback, individuals and organizations can ensure that the highest quality of affordable service is being supplied.

Risk management involves the identification of potential problems and how these might be anticipated and avoided. If an adverse event occurs, structures should be in place to be able to rapidly detect it, investigate it and alter existing practice to prevent its recurrence.

To establish whether the guidelines for best clinical practice are being followed, *clinical audit* should be an integral part of a unit or individual's development. Audit is related to evidence-based medicine, provision of a quality service and research. Departmental audit is a contractual requirement for ophthalmologists and personal audit should be considered in the same light. Every surgeon should be aware of the quality outcome measures of each quantifiable area of his or her clinical practice. This will allow a more accurate prognosis to be given to the patient preoperatively. It will also demonstrate the surgeon's constant commitment to high quality clinical performance if challenged in a court of law.

Certain aspects of ophthalmological practice lend themselves to clinical audit as they are readily identifiable and quantifiable outcome measures. In cataract surgery the two outcome measures that are easiest to audit are visual acuity improvement, from pre- to postoperative, and rates of posterior capsular rupture. Individuals and departments should have the data collection mechanisms in place to be able to review current practice on a regular basis. You can use the information to drive your individual learning cycle and departmental performance.

Chapter 9

Medicolegal matters

COMMUNICATION AND THE DOCTOR–PATIENT RELATIONSHIP

Good communication is the basis for the development of any important relationship. Patients place an enormous trust in their surgeon and this should not be taken lightly. What may seem to you a routine cataract is a very special problem for that patient (how many times have you been told by a patient that 'your eyesight is precious'?). Trust is nurtured and enhanced by a friendly approach and an open two-way consultation. Within the confines of the clinic, it is up to the doctor to create the feeling that each patient is special and each patient's problem is important.

The patient attending for the first time will be nervous and apprehensive about the outcome of the consultation. Efforts to create a relaxed environment will encourage the patient to give a more comprehensive history, which might be crucial in future management plans. A handshake, a smile and eye contact can all be achieved within the first few seconds of any consultation but their effects may last for years to come. If the relationship is cultivated and nurtured, a firm bond will be established which will help both individuals if complications ensue.

Patients cite a physician's ability to listen and empathize as two of the most important attributes. It has been estimated that although it takes a patient an average of 60 seconds to summarize their chief complaint, about three-quarters of doctors will interrupt within 20 seconds! It may be prudent to afford the patient and yourself that extra 40 seconds of clinic time.

Similarly, the manner in which you approach the patient after a surgical complication will determine the course of the doctor–patient relationship in the postoperative period. The atmosphere in the operating theatre and the way news is broken the following day will be crucial for further consultations. The patient will almost certainly need further medical care, and hard as it will seem at the time, the patient has to be kept on-side and involved.

The population as a whole is better educated, and one of the consequences of that education is the readiness to consider litigation for any adverse medical event. Solicitors now actively advertise within and without hospitals, looking to 'help' patients achieve redress for misadventure. Surgeons must be aware of the potential for legal action at every turn. Experience suggests that litigation is best avoided or moderated by the instigation of risk-reduction strategies, i.e. by pursuing and demonstrating that you have pursued best practice. This may seem like a counsel of perfection, but really is not difficult.

DEFENSIVE STRATEGIES

Medical records

A surgeon is challenged to be thorough in his or her management of a patient and to demonstrate that thoroughness. A medical record of the highest standards is compelling evidence of that quality of care. Auditing of surgery is easier and problems can be fully reviewed. If a case comes to review as part of a legal process, well kept, complete and thorough notes will greatly help all concerned. They will reflect well on the surgeon and provide clear evidence of the quality of care offered to that patient. Explanations are easier, apologies more likely to be accepted, and litigation to be defended. The converse is also true and an incomplete set of notes, with unintelligible abbreviations and inconsistencies, will reflect badly.

With the advent of electronic data handling systems, the emphasis will move away from the production of well-written, complete medical records. At present, however, these documents remain as an indelible record of the care given to individual patients. The quality of medical notes can be used in your defence and prevent a downfall if a case comes to court.

Practical note-keeping

The habitual recording of the patient's history and symptoms (i.e. the justification for surgery) and all positive and negative physical signs in the examination is crucial. Care should be given to record the visual acuity, refraction, pupillary reactions, lid cleanliness, endothelial signs, the presence or absence of pseudoexfoliation, lens stability, cataract morphology, intraocular pressure and the retinal findings through the dilated pupil.

The operative record can be done either longhand or by completing a tick sheet (Fig. 9.1). The sheet should have boxes for the alternative steps needed for some operations. A full, contemporary description of any complication must be given in either longhand or dictated. This may feel rather risky, but revealing anything less than the full circumstances will increase concern about the integrity of the record when peer-reviewed. More questions will follow and doubts increase.

The postoperative recovery and progress should be charted and any adverse events fully recorded, together with a note of investigations and the treatments undertaken or offered. If there has been a complication, record any conversations with the patient and relatives and outline what was said and by whom.

The surgery must be seen, or 'read', to have been complete. An operation note that reads simply 'routine phaco – no complications' will probably be sufficient for an intradepartmental audit as the surgeon's general 'routine' practice will be known, i.e. what sort of section, the technique for phacoemulsification and any antibiotic prophylaxis. In a courtroom with aggressive strangers the situation is different. You may be asked 'How did you prepare the eye preoperatively?' in a case of postoperative endophthalmitis. You may routinely use povidine-iodine wash but unless the operative note actually states that, you will be challenged: 'Did you actually use this solution in this case or did you forget?'.

Quality of the written record

The standard of note-keeping reflects the standard of care offered by a surgical team, and the culture of an eye department. What may be acceptable brevity in note-keeping when working single-handed in the bush, is an inadequate standard for a patient looked after in a teaching hospital department. It is tempting to take short cuts when writing notes for such repetitive conditions as cataract or recording its routine surgery, but this is where problems can begin if complications occur.

The medical record is a vital document and the strongest objective evidence to an outsider of how well you look after your patients. Imagine yourself being scrutinized as

---

Box 9.1 Questions to ask yourself about the notes you have made

▶ Are they legible?
▶ Is the record complete?
▶ Is it obvious that your examination looked for potentially complicating factors, e.g. corneal guttata, pseudoexfoliation?
▶ Did the patient actually have a cataract that required surgery?
▶ Why was surgery done, for example, to improve vision or reduce glare?
▶ Is it apparent that appropriate care was taken if such problems were anticipated?
▶ Who was present at the time of surgery?
▶ Do your notes clearly and openly describe what happened and how any complication was handled?
▶ Is the note signed with a legible signature?

---

part of a medicolegal process; it will certainly focus your mind!

Abbreviations or shorthand should be kept to a minimum; they are open to misinterpretation and what may be easily understood by the person who writes the abbreviation may be unintelligible to other members of a surgical firm not intimately associated with the day-to-day running of the surgery. Later generations of doctors may have no idea of what an abbreviation may mean, for example does 'N.A.D.' mean 'No Abnormality Detected' or 'Not Actually Done'?

A good impression is given by recording negative as well as positive findings. It shows that potential problems were looked for, even if not found. For example, in the case of a patient whose lens is lost into the vitreous, by recording that preoperatively there was no evidence of pseudoexfoliation, the surgeon was not expected to take more than a normal amount of care with the capsule/zonule. If some abnormality is seen preoperatively the surgeon must demonstrate that the appropriate extra care was taken. The converse is obviously also true, that a poorly written and incomplete record of your examination, for example failing to record the presence or absence of signs of pseudoexfoliation, will indicate that a less than studied approach had been taken to the patient's eyes in the preoperative assessment.

Similarly, when writing operation notes, record simply the routine steps in the operation. This will underline the standard of care you gave that patient. For instance, in a patient in whom endophthalmitis later develops, by recording that you carefully cleaned the lids with antiseptic wash, draped the lids and gave the patient postopera-

THE LEEDS TEACHING HOSPITALS	Eye Department **Operative Report**	

Sticker

Patient's Name .... Date ....

Patient's Address ....

....

Date of Birth ....Hospital No ....

Consultant ....Ward .... Surgeon ....

DC/ONS	GA/LA	

Operation: ☐ Phacoemulsification + IOL ☐ Extracapsular Extraction + IOL ☐ Other *(see over)*

Preparation:	☐ Povidone-iodine	☐ Other ....
	☐ Wire lid speculum	☐ Superior Rectus suture ☐ Inferior Rectus suture

Entry: ☐ Posterior corneal ☐ Phaco tunnel ☐ Other ....

Anterior Capsulotomy: ☐ Capsulorhexis ☐ Letter box ☐ Other ....

Comments ....

Nucleus:	☐ Expression	☐ Phaco Technique: Divide + Conquer
	☐ Phacoemulsification	☐ Phaco Chop ☐ Other ....

Cortical Aspiration:		**Phaco Time:**
	☐ Manual	☐ Simcoe
	☐ Auto	☐ McIntyre

Capsule Polishing: ☐ Manual ☐ Auto

Lens Implantation: ☐ Bag ☐ Sulcus

☐ Other ....

Affix IOL Sticker Here

Wound Closure: ☐ Running ☐ Interrupted ☐ None

☐ 10/0 nylon   Other ....

Intraocular Fluids:	☐ BSS 500mls	☐ with 0.5mg Adrenalin
	☐ Healonid	☐ Acetycholine
	☐ Other viscoelastic	

Subconj: ☐ Betnesol 2mg ☐ Cefuroxime 125mg ☐ Gentamicin 20mg

Topical Drops:

Complications: Yes ☐ No ☐ *(see over)*

Signed: ....

To be completed after operative procedure by scrub nurse

Specimens noted in register Yes ☐ No ☐

Details of drains, catheters, pack etc ....

....

Count correct .... Signed ....

Operation Note:	**Date:**

Surgeon:

Assistant:

Signed: ....

Specimens noted in register Yes ☐ No ☐

Details of drains, catheters, pack etc ....

....

Count correct .... Signed ....

Fig. 9.1 Tick sheet as an operative record

tive antibiotic drops in theatre will indicate that all reasonable steps had been taken to try to prevent infection. Defensive treatment and defensive recording of that treatment underlines the quality of the care given to that patient. It is much easier to defend this situation.

Finally, all notes must be signed and dated by the inscriber. Junior doctors come and go and the identification of a given physician from an illegible initial can prove very frustrating in years to come. All staff, including consultants, should be encouraged to either print their names under their signature or to use a personalized stamp.

MANAGING A COMPLICATION IN THEATRE

The atmosphere in the operating theatre should be calm and quiet. When teaching or learning, all criticisms or problem discussions should be reserved for the coffee room and not gratuitously dispensed in front of the patient. Remember that a patient's memory of the actual words spoken will blur with time, such that the word 'problem' could become interpreted as 'disaster'.

Talk quietly and with circumspection. Use neutral words and keep the tone of the voice even, even if your heart is racing as the operative plan falls apart. Tell the patient that 'this might take a little longer' and they will relax, knowing that the matter is safe in your hands. During the operation, it is important to talk quietly and think before speaking, especially when dealing with a complication.

Music in theatre should be sensitively chosen; loud pop music, which may be sweet to your ears, will grate in the ears of an 80-year-old.

When teaching, it is well worth agreeing a 'code' of phases that will be used, for example, 'would you like me to do this bit' actually means 'I want to take over'. Every word is listened to and criticisms should be avoided. It is important to save comment until after the operation is complete. Review of a complication immediately after the surgery, perhaps looking at a video recording of the operation, allows for critique away from the ears of the patient and will be less threatening for the trainee.

POSTOPERATIVE EXPLANATIONS

The way in which an issue is handled will do much to mollify the patient and their relatives. Careful, quiet, timely explanations will immediately inform the patient and bring them into the discussion about the problem, its management and expected outcome. They are thus effectively included in the therapeutic effort and their confidence and trust will be maintained (see Box 9.2).

Box 9.2 When and what to say following a complicated operation

► A short explanation should be given immediately after the operation. The scene is set for the next day and patient and family are prepared for a fuller explanation. This will be easier if the patient was carefully warned in the preoperative period of any anticipated problems, e.g. pseudoexfoliation

► Repeat the explanation, but in full, the following day. Not all that you say will be remembered or understood. It is therefore useful to invite the patient to bring a relative or friend to the next and subsequent visits to help the family understand what has happened. This openness brings another pair of ears to hear your explanation and may be very useful in encouraging the patient to continue, start *and* complete the treatment course outlined

► Repeat and explain the problems (and be prepared to re-explain the matter) at subsequent appointments

► Remember that careless talk can cause later problems. Misjudged exclamations in the operating theatre, especially when the going gets tough, should be avoided

► Trainers should be moderate in what they say or they will tend to cause more problems than they help

---

At present, doctors in the UK are not legally obliged to provide patients with an explanation after complicated surgery. This is not the case in some other countries, for example Canada. In a recent study, over 80% of patients felt that a patient should always be told if a complication has occurred and the possible adverse outcomes that might ensue. Only 33% of ophthalmologists felt the same way. The medicolegal issues that surround this area are explored later in this chapter.

MEDICOLEGAL MATTERS

A complication may or may not be negligent. What will make it negligent is the way it is responded to or handled.

The concept of defensive surgery was introduced earlier in the book. Paranoia and over-confidence (arrogance?) represent either end of the spectrum of a doctor's attitude towards a patient. Erring towards the former extreme is a prudent precaution in these more litigious times. The patient's consent distinguishes a surgical procedure from an assault. Even with informed consent, some patients may sue their physician following a complication of treatment. Some surgical complications are associated with more frequent negligence claims than others. Considering all claims, some suggestions can be made with regard to risk-reduction strategies.

THE LITIGIOUS PATIENT

There is no defining characteristic that identifies the patient who will sue, but there is one emotion that links all litigious patients and that is anger. Most patients seek medical care because they want to be cured not because they are thinking of suing. With the recent advances in medical care, patients not only want to be cured, they expect to be cured. When these expectations are not realized some will seek litigation as redress. Surprise at a poorer than expected outcome may turn to anger if communication between the surgeon and patient is poor or avoided.

Good patient education in the preoperative work-up is the physician's chance to ground expectation in realism.

If a complication occurs, the doctor–patient relationship will be tested. The stronger it is the better the chance of helping the patient over a difficult period. If there are problems and issues that cannot be rapidly resolved, it is often best to pre-empt matters and offer the patient a second opinion with another expert. Time should be set aside which can be devoted to postoperative counselling. The patient should be seen regularly by the most senior member of the team in clinic. Openness and honesty will foster trust.

WHICH CASES END UP IN COURT?

Any problem that results in a less than perfect functional and cosmetic result can generate a medicolegal claim. Most litigation following cataract surgery is due to mistakes with the IOL. Inaccurate biometry, failing to take into account the refractive state of the fellow eye and problems reading the computer print-out, can all lead to the wrong power being used. This may require a contact lens, refractive surgery, 'piggybacking' or IOL exchange to correct. Decentration or malposition of an IOL can cause just as many subjective problems.

Other complications can result in legal proceedings but the most common are those which lead to a poorer visual outcome. These will include a ruptured posterior capsule, vitreous loss and retained lens material. Expulsive haemorrhage and endophthalmitis are the complications we most fear as they result in the worst visual outcome or even loss of an eye.

Provided the patient did not have uncontrolled hypertension or poor blood clotting secondary to warfarin, suprachoroidal haemorrhage is easy to defend and few of the ensuing problems can be attributed to the surgeon.

Conversely, endophthalmitis cases are usually the most expensive as it is easier to blame the surgeon for lack of

vigilance or incomplete pre- and postoperative management. The usual complaint in these cases is that while postoperative inflammation was noted, it was not aggressively investigated or treated.

RISK-REDUCTION STRATEGIES

A well-managed complication should result in a good visual outcome and litigation is less likely. There are some management strategies and protocols that can be followed which reduce the risk of an adverse event and subsequent litigation. Some of these strategies can be applied to all ophthalmic procedures and some are specifically for cataract surgery. These are set out in Boxes 9.3 and 9.4 respectively.

Box 9.3 General ophthalmic risk-reduction

▶ Fully document the preoperative examination, especially noting positive and negative findings which may affect outcome, and the indications for surgery

▶ Document the discussion concerning risks of surgery and prognosis

▶ Indicate if an education sheet/booklet has been given to the patient

▶ Obtain informed consent – the use of an operation-specific consent form will help

▶ Write or dictate a complete operative report. This should include any steps to prevent infection (povidine wash, intracameral or postoperative antibiotics), the description of any complication and the steps taken to manage it and the reasons for choosing a particular IOL power and style. Document the absence of complications and the use of various preparations, no matter how routine

▶ Take all patients' concerns seriously after the operation

▶ Manage all flashes, floaters, pain and visual deterioration aggressively

▶ Afford more time to follow up patients who are angry or aggrieved. Discussions with these people should be thoroughly documented and, preferably, witnessed

▶ Never make any changes to a previous record on the basis of belatedly observed findings

▶ Ask for senior advice or a second opinion early

Box 9.4 Risk-reduction in cataract surgery

► Ensure technicians or nurses who perform biometry are well trained
► Review the A-scans and other data yourself
► Use a third generation formula for IOL power calculation
► Use a limited number of IOL styles to prevent confusion, and have their A-constants pinned to the side of the cabinet
► Clearly mark the IOL power and style on an operating list in the theatre – either on a white board or on paper
► Do not operate beyond your experience, e.g. don't try to remove a dropped nuclear fragment or attempt a complicated lens implant unless you have been shown how

The importance of good communication cannot be stressed enough. It is the fundamental strategy to reduce risk. The patient must be able to ask and be told about their condition in a manner that they can understand. The explanation must be comprehensive and appropriate. Document your care of the case and the patient's concerns. Remember that your well-kept medical records should be your best ally if things go wrong and that the converse is also true, that poorly kept notes will become your worst enemy.

A recurring factor in the cascade of issues that lead to a patient seeking redress for injury, whether surgical or medical, is the breakdown of the doctor–patient relationship. Failure to explain simply, clearly and in a timely way what has happened undermines the trust the patient has placed in the doctor. Failure to tell the patient of a complication is poorly perceived, aggravates the problem and invites anger and a search for an apology or financial settlement in court. The chances of being sued are increased by any lack of honesty or openness by the clinician.

Bibliography

Beatty S, Lotery A, Kent D, O'Driscoll A, Kilmartin DJ, Wallace D, Baglivo E (1998) Acute intraoperative suprachoroidal haemorrhage in ocular surgery. *Eye* 12 (5): 815–20.

Brick DC (1999) Risk management lessons from a review of 168 cataract surgery claims. *Surv Ophthalmol* 43 (4): 356–60.

Charlton J and Weinstein G (1995) *Ophthalmic Surgery Complications.* Philadelphia: Lippincott, pp. 95–115.

Desai P, Minassian DC and Reidy A (1999) National cataract surgery survey 1997–8: a report of the results of the clinical outcomes. *Br J Ophthalmol* 83: 1336–40.

Desai P, Reidy A and Minassian DC (1999) Profile of patients presenting for cataract surgery in the UK: national data collection. *Br J Ophthalmol* 83: 893–6.

Hingorani M, Wong T and Vafidis G (1999) Patients' and doctors' attitudes to amount of information given after unintended injury during treatment: cross sectional, questionnaire survey. *Br Med J* 318: 640–1.

Koch PS (1992) *Converting to Phacoemulsification,* 3rd edn. New York: Slack.

Koch PS (1997) *Simplifying Phacoemulsification: Safe and Efficient Methods for Cataract Surgery,* 5th edn. New York: Slack.

Kraff CR and Kraff MC (1999) Cataract surgery. In Krupin T, Kolker A and Rosenberg L (eds), *Complications in Ophthalmic Surgery,* 2nd edn. St Louis: Mosby, pp. 57–77.

Kraushar MF (1992) Recognizing and managing the litigious patient. *Surv Ophthalmol* 37 (1): 54–6.

Seibel BS (1999) *Phacodynamics: Mastering the Tools and Techniques of Phacoemulsification Surgery,* 3rd edn. New York: Slack.

Index

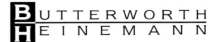
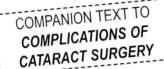
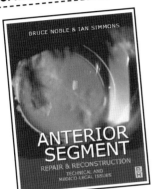
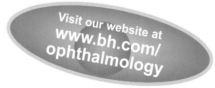